TRANSACTIONS OF THE

AMERICAN PHILOSOPHICAL SOCIETY

HELD AT PHILADELPHIA

FOR PROMOTING USEFUL KNOWLEDGE

VOLUME 67, PART 3 · 1977

Medicine and Society in Tanganyika 1890–1930

A Historical Inquiry

ANN BECK

PROFESSOR EMERITUS OF HISTORY, UNIVERSITY OF HARTFORD

THE AMERICAN PHILOSOPHICAL SOCIETY

INDEPENDENCE SQUARE: PHILADELPHIA

April, 1977

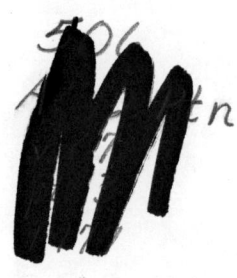

To
RONALD and MEREDITH
LINKS WITH THE FUTURE

Copyright © 1977 by The American Philosophical Society
Library of Congress Catalog
Card Number 76-50176
International Standard Book Number 0-87169-673-8
US ISSN 0065-9746

ACKNOWLEDGMENTS

This work was in part supported by NIH Grant LM 26,411 from the National Library of Medicine. Support by the American Philosophical Society enabled me to travel to the German Archives in Potsdam in 1974. I gratefully acknowledge the help I received.

Several government archives and university libraries permitted me to study documents and other materials without which this monograph could not have progressed beyond the stage of incomplete reporting. I am particularly indebted to the archivist and librarian of the Zentrale Staatsarchiv in Potsdam, D. D. R., for granting me access to valuable material on the social, administrative, and medical background of colonial Tanganyika. The National Archives in Dar es Salaam permitted me to study relevant documents in their collections of the old German files. The German Archives in Koblenz, F. D. R., provided access to the papers of leading colonial officials who contributed to the making of colonial history between 1890 and 1918. At the Bernhard-Nocht-Institut für Schiffs- und- Tropenkrankheiten in Hamburg I read leading medical journals which had survived the destruction of World War II. The Library of Yale University enabled me to read many issues of colonial journals, newspapers and books published before 1918.

The listing of names of institutions may be tedious to the reader but to the historian they represent the life line that connects him with the past. My thanks go to the many officials, archivists, librarians, and historians whom I met in the course of the preparation of this study.

GLOSSARY AND ABBREVIATIONS

Akida	Arab or African administrator in charge of several subdistricts but always responsible to his superior German official.
Arbeiterfrage	Term used throughout the colonial period to describe the difficulties of labor recruitment and the shortage of farm workers on European plantations. Translated as "labor problem."
Bezirksamt	District office for administrative and legislative matters relating to Africans.
DKG	Deutsche Kolonialgesellschaft (German Colonial Society)
DOAG	Deutsch-Ostafrika Gesellschaft (German East African Company)
KWK	Kolonialwirtschaftliches Komitee (Colonial Economic Committee) established for the general improvement of the Protectorate and especially for the production of raw materials in DOA and the sale of German manufactured goods in the colony.
Jumbe	Village headman or chief
Maji Maji	Swahili for Water Water. The term was used as a rallying cry during the revolt in the Southern Highlands in 1905–1906.
Regierungsarzt	Physician employed by the civilian administration in contrast to the sanitation staff officer of the Schutztruppe.
Reichsgesundheitsamt	Imperial Ministry of Health
Reichskommissar	Highest official in the colony before the appointment of governors.
Schutztruppe	German military force during the colonial period.
TNA	Tanzania National Archives

MEDICINE AND SOCIETY IN TANGANYIKA, 1890–1930; A HISTORICAL INQUIRY

ANN BECK

CONTENTS

	PAGE
Introductory remarks	5
I. The historical setting of German East Africa	5
II. Western medicine and German East Africa: a start	9
III. Colonial policy and malaria control in German East Africa	13
IV. Sleeping sickness in German East Africa: scientific experiments and political expediencies	17
V. Social policy in German East Africa: public health, medicine, and the labor question	22
VI. Medicine, science, and society toward the end of German rule in East Africa	28
VII. World War I and its impact on people, politics, and health	37
VIII. Concluding essay	46
Appendix:	
I. Comments on statistics	50
II. Selected documents	50
Bibliography	55
Index	57

INTRODUCTORY REMARKS

The central role which medicine was destined to play in colonial territories was recognized from the very beginning but it took a long time until colonial governments gave medical departments adequate priority within the system. It was not a lack of fighting spirit or conviction on the part of medical administrators which assigned the role of Cinderella to the medical departments. Colonial governments were exposed to pressures by diplomats, business interests, agricultural settlers, and patriotic societies at all times and in the course of conflicting interests the most urgent health requirements were not given the attention they deserved. For many years, therefore, after German colonial government had been established in East Africa, large numbers of peasants in the vast stretches of the colony remained exposed to the dangers threatening them in their tropical environment.

This book traces the growth of the colonial medical services in German East Africa and shows the obstacles they met in the course of the years. Although non-political by definition, the medical department was subjected to influences far transcending its own sphere. Its development offers to the historian a unique opportunity to explore the cross-currents of colonial history. The story of the German East African medical administration and its continuation under the British Mandate in 1919 is presented here as a contribution to the history of Tanganyika as a whole.* Both the German and the British phases in Tanganyika share many common characteristics in spite of differences in detail and in their approach to African society as such.

The similarity of primary factors which influenced disease and health such as geography, climate, and biological conditions, prescribed the basic goals of medical administrators in Tanganyika under German and English rule. But differences in political tradition and styles of life in their home countries influenced the conduct of an otherwise predetermined task. In this way an analysis of the social role performed by the German and British medical services in Tanganyika uncovers some of the complexities of colonial East African development. It is hoped that the use of new documentary material, only recently available to the historian, has added novelty to the treatment of a controversial theme in colonial history.

I. THE HISTORICAL SETTING OF GERMAN EAST AFRICA

When the German government gave protection to the German Society for Colonization in 1885 and placed the Society's territories under the sovereignty of the German Reich, German imperial involvement on African soil had begun.[1] When Herrmann von Wissmann was appointed imperial commissioner for German East Africa in 1888 and added two doctors to his staff, a beginning was made of an imperial medical service in the newly acquired East African colony. Before that time medical matters had been the responsibility of individuals who suffered severely because of their lack of knowledge of the major tropical diseases. Malaria and dysentery were described as scourges by those who ventured into the East African interior. As accidents occurred frequently on expeditions, the survival of travelers and explorers was a matter of sheer luck as long as they lacked professional help.[2]

Though fully aware of the fact that health was vital for the success of missionary enterprises, commercial ventures, and scientific expeditions, it was not included

---

* For examples of the literature see appended bibliography.

[1] Reginald Coupland, *East Africa and Its Invaders from its Earliest Times to the Death of Seyyid Said in 1856* (Oxford, 1938) and Coupland, *The Exploitation of East Africa, 1856–1890* (London, 1939).

[2] See particularly Wilhelm Langheld, *Zwanzig Jahre in deutschen Kolonien* (Berlin, 1909), pp. 94 and 95. Rochus Schmidt, *Geschichte des Araberaufstandes in Ost-Afrika* (Frankfurt/Oder, 1892), pp. 258–259. Idem, *Aus Kolonialer Frühzeit* (Berlin, 1939), pp. 104–105.

in the advance planning of those who ventured into the interior. It seems that the early adventurers and travelers were possessed by a fatalism matched only by that of the practitioners of witchcraft. Even when colonial operations began to be better organized in the 1880's, priority was given to the "pacification" and the effective establishment of local control. It is this preoccupation with military operations during the early German administrations which influenced German attitudes toward colonial medical policy and determined its course for many years thereafter.

To the modern observer it is puzzling to find in official and unofficial German reports for the period many statements which repeatedly stressed that the promotion of medicine and public health was vital to the development of German East Africa (*Deutsch Ostafrika*, DOA). But as late as 1910 ten million inhabitants in DOA had only forty-three doctors to look after their needs. And of this number thirty-six doctors were employed by the government and therefore burdened with administrative as well as purely medical work.[3] Also in 1910 a startling statement by Colonial Secretary Bernard Dernburg surprises the modern reader. He wrote, "A system of medical care for the blacks, even in the government sector of the medical services, does not yet exist. The introduction of such a system is our goal although the means to secure it will probably surpass the present capability of the protectorate."[4] On the other hand, great achievements in the control of tropical diseases were made and medical as well as scientific research had reached a respectable level in the colony by 1914. How does one explain these contradictions? The reexamination of the causes of these apparent inconsistencies leads the historian to an analysis of colonial policy as such. A brief historical introduction precedes, therefore, the presentation of medical and social developments. Its aim is solely to place the socio-medical events of the early colonial period in proper perspective.

On the eve of the partition of East Africa in the 1880's the British had established themselves as the leading European power in Zanzibar but their position was tenuous. It depended very much on the absence of competing European intruders. Moreover, British influence extended primarily to Zanzibar and was not felt in the interior. The British had not attempted to assume administrative functions in the port towns or further inland. Nor did the British government find it necessary to subsidize or protect British traders before 1888.[5] The success of British cooperation with the sultan of Zanzibar hinged on the ability of the British consul to maintain the appearance of the sultan's independence, and to give moral support to his claim of exercising sovereignty over the interior of East Africa where neither his name nor his power played a leading role. In their dealings with Zanzibar the British were primarily motivated by two objectives. One was the restriction and eventual abolition of the slave trade, and the second was the expansion of imports from India and England to East Africa as well as the export of tropical goods from East Africa to Europe. Consul Kirk had repeatedly urged the British government to support a chartered company in one of the port towns but he had not received any favorable response prior to the "scramble" of 1885 which led to open competition of the European powers for control of east and central Africa. In 1884 the era of British remote control of Zanzibar politics had come to an end. A new type of conquistador arrived on the scene. It would be misleading, however, to interpret British predominance in Zanzibar during the first three-quarters of the nineteenth century as evidence of an exclusively Arab-British condominium. Zanzibar and its hinterland had been open to scientists, geographers, philanthropists, missionaries, and small-scale traders and adventurers from the western world before and after Livingstone.

The history of German contacts with East Africa in the nineteenth century differs essentially from that of their British predecessors. As early as 1859 two large Hamburg business concerns, O'Swald and Hansing, had established trade relations with Zanzibar.[6] They were able to invest considerable capital and weathered the obstacles of slow returns on profits, the high cost of transportation, and the losses through long-term credits extended to Indian merchants in East Africa. But they were not the only representatives of German interests in the area. After the unification of Germany in 1871 a new type of political adventurer arrived. Inexperienced and unconcerned with the safety of their economic investment, they were primarily motivated politically. They wanted a foothold in East Africa for Germany to match the previous advances made by England and France. To this group belonged Dr. Karl Peters who founded the German Society for Colonization in Berlin in 1884.[7] His associates in this venture

---

[3] Z St A, Potsdam, R Kol A no 1026, Bl 90–91, 15 August, 1910.

[4] Z St A, Potsdam, R Kol A no 1024, Bl 12.

[5] A British captain, W. F. Owen, had hoisted the British flag from 1824 to 1826 in Mombasa in support of its ruling family, the Mazrui. The Foreign Office in London ordered Owen to abstain from taking sides in the struggle between Mombasa and Zanzibar. See Coupland, *East Africa and Its Invaders*, p. 168, and Franz Ferdinand Müller, *Deutschland-Zanzibar-Ostafrika* (Berlin, 1959), pp. 72, 73.

[6] Coupland, *The Exploitation of East Africa*, p. 303.

[7] A detailed account of Peters's aspirations cannot be given in the context of this chapter. Contemporary writers as well as recent historians agree that he was a rabid nationalist and that his motives were primarily political. He wanted to make Germany a leading colonial power. His demagogic expostulations annoyed even many of his contemporaries who shared his expansionist views. The German explorer Georg Schweinfurth referred to Peters's actions as "colonial hooliganism." (Schweinfurth to Dr. Paul Kayser, director of the Colonial Division of the German Foreign Office, 18 March, 1896. Bundesarchiv, Koblenz, *Kleine Erwerbungen*, No. 10, 18 March, 1896.) See also Müller, *op. cit.*, pp. 99–114. It is significant that

were Graf Felix Behr, a conservative aristocrat, and Friedrich Lange, a nationalistic journalist. Peters was impressed by his observation of British imperial politics during visits to England and was disappointed by the absence of an active colonial policy in Germany. He therefore decided to bring about a change of attitude which would involve German officials in an aggressive colonial policy. He presented his country with a *fait accompli* after he had collected sufficient funds for a hurried expedition to Zanzibar in September of 1884. Together with Dr. Karl Jühlke, Count Joachim Pfeil, and merchant August Otto, he went to East Africa where, within three weeks, he succeeded in concluding twelve treaties with Arab and African chiefs who were not aware of the extent of territory they were giving to the German colonization society.[8] The territory was estimated as covering 2,500 square miles and was of strategic value since it was on the mainland west of Zanzibar and close enough to the island to allow for trade.[9] After his return to Germany, Peters lobbied for imperial support of his commercial paper empire and succeeded in receiving an imperial charter (*Schutzbrief*) for his company in 1885. And it did not take long before the protective power given to German individuals was extended to representatives of the German Reich. The next step after this start was the dispatch of a protective armed force to the African mainland by the German emperor. The German East African Protectorate had been born.[10]

By 1890 the political map of East Africa shows a clearly delineated German colony with political boundaries agreed upon in treaties between England, Germany, and the sultan of Zanzibar who relinquished his claim to the coast. German East Africa reached to Lake Victoria in the west and to the Rovuma River and Lake Nyasa in the south.

After the unprecedented speed of the earlier developments, the difficult task of establishing a viable administration began. The Germans faced a country whose previous European invaders had been prospectors, anti-slavery apostles, and scientists. It had not been settled by westerners nor did the German intruders know how the African peoples would react to the foreign take-over. Besides, the Germans were ignorant about Arab and Swahili officials with whom they must come to terms.

In establishing control over DOA the Germans did not follow a predetermined policy. Developments occurred as the result of shifting diplomatic events in Europe in the 1880's. At the same time the government reacted to pressures from within on an *ad hoc* basis, first in dealing with Dr. Peters, then in making concessions to the Society for German Colonization and finally in reaching agreements with the German East Africa Company and its attempts to shape public opinion. In spite of these uncertainties important precedents were set between 1885 and 1890. Promises were made and interest groups established which continued to claim special privileges as their legally valid rights later on. Two of the most vocal companies during the earlier years were the German Colonial Society (*Deutsche Kolonialgesellschaft,* DKG) and the German East Africa Company (*Deutsch Ostafrika Kompanie,* DOAK). The latter complained bitterly in 1892 that its contract, concluded with the government in November, 1890, had not been kept. Among others the government had promised a close and intimate cooperation with the company and had offered to submit all government measures relating to the economic development in East Africa to the company's approval prior to the implementation of such measures in the colony.[11] Similarly the planters referred for many years to privileges they considered themselves entitled to under the terms of their settlement in DOA. All these assumptions were woven into an image which formed the basis of the future relationship between the government and the private sector in East Africa.

The accidental and makeshift character of the initial stages of colonial administration was felt and expressed by several of the men who served in the colony during various periods. Oskar Karstedt, for instance, a district commissioner in Ujiji in 1910, wrote in his reminiscences that Germany took a leap into Africa without really knowing what it involved. "When Germany entered the ranks of the active colonial powers," he wrote, "it had to face problems which it was not prepared to solve as yet as far as its personnel, its material capacity and its scientific preparedness were concerned."[12] He cited the unfamiliarity by legal advisers (*Assessoren*) with conditions in Africa, the lieutenants' lack of experience of how to deal with an African recruit, the medical men's lack of experience of malaria and blackwater fever and the farmers' lack of knowledge of tropical conditions. Scientists and explorers who had been in Africa, he wrote, were of no use for the purpose of opening up colonization in Africa. And Theodor Gunzert, a district commissioner in Mwanza from 1907 to 1916, wrote in retrospect that Germany's foundation of a colonial empire was a leap into the darkness. East Africa was unknown to the Germans except as a place for trade in slaves and

---

with Peters the center of operations shifted from the more cosmopolitan Hamburg to the new capital of the German Reich in Berlin.

[8] Jühlke and Pfeil came from well-to-do middle-class families. Not tied to a position or a profession, they could plunge into the East African venture readily. Müller, *op. cit.,* p. 104.

[9] Coupland, *Exploitation of East Africa,* p. 401; Scott Keltie, *The Partition of Africa* (London, 1893), p. 229.

[10] Bismarck delayed the granting of a charter until the conclusion of the Berlin Conference.

[11] Z St A, Potsdam, R Kol A, no. 764, Bl 111–119, 23 October, 1892, and *ibid.* no. 118, Bl 3, 8, 14.

[12] Oskar Karstedt, *Der Weisse Kampf um Afrika* 2 (Berlin, 1938): p. 60.

ivory.[13] Although the two men served in East Africa before 1900, they had become aware of the unsound basis of the colonial administration during its early years. The German start in East Africa was amateurish. By 1887 Dr. Peters was removed as head of the German East Africa Company. Moreover, relations with Zanzibar changed when Sultan Khalifa succeeded Sultan Barghash. A new treaty in 1888 granted the company total control over its economic sphere of influence on the mainland.[14]

New complications arose. Arab and Swahili resistance developed to the German representatives of the company and led to drastic military action. The Arab leader Bushiri who held out longer than others was hanged. The suppression of the Arab revolt by German military and naval action had far reaching results. A military police force under Herrmann von Wissmann was sent to East Africa to "pacify" the country and declared its mission completed by 1890 but the precedent thus created had lasting repercussions on the future civilian and medical administrations of the country.

Wissmann seemed to be the right man for the appointment as imperial commissioner (*Reichskommissar*) in 1888. His military experience in the regular army and his participation in several African expeditions qualified him for the new job. He had formed very definite views on the destructive results of the slave trade in the Congo and wrote after his expedition in 1885,

the responsibility of having caused these evils [the destruction of formerly flourishing villages] rests without question with the Arabs, for only through their initiative was it possible to penetrate further, to subject still more people and to depopulate [the country], and therefore, if one wants to help the poor natives, the Arabs in these territories must be eradicated totally."[15]

His anti-Arab sentiments and a paternalistic sympathy with the "poor natives" can be discerned in his policy during his tenure in the colony. Wissmann's budget was limited to two million marks and his military force of twenty-one officers, a few civilian officials and doctors in addition to forty-two sergeants and a striking force made up of Sudanese, Zulu, and Somali could not cover the vast area which he was to pacify and organize.[16] The *Schutztruppe* accomplished its task. The German flag replaced that of the sultan along the coast, a new station, Moshi, was opened up in the interior, the sultan sold his East African possessions for four million marks, and the German East African Protectorate was ready to begin its administration.

Wissmann's achievements between 1888 and 1890 have been the subject of controversial evaluations. His close associates admired him as a great soldier. Wissmann himself wrote, in his final report to the government, "the East African coast has been reconquered and its possession has been secured by the erection of fortifications and lines of communications so that the latter [the coast] can be secured against all eventualities with a relatively very small contingent of troops."[17] As an administrator the imperial commissioner has been subjected to considerable criticism. Michahelles, the German consul general in Zanzibar, wrote in a private letter on March 5, 1890, "a military dictatorship, as practiced by Wissmann today, has no value in the long run; as soon as the South has been occupied, a definite organization will have to be introduced as soon as possible." He criticized the cursory hanging of Arabs as impractical because it deprived the Germans of the potentially most useful reservoir of lower-echelon administrators. The continuation of a state of emergency would make it difficult to reestablish normal conditions and he concluded that for the reorganization of the colony a high ranking official would have to be installed in Zanzibar who would assume political control over all diverse interests.[18] Bismarck seems to have shared this view. He replaced Wissmann with Count von Soden who had served as governor in the Cameroons before coming to Zanzibar in 1891.

During the early years of German rule in East Africa harsh military policies and occasional ruthless campaigns to suppress local resistance existed side by side with the determination to develop contact with Africans and Arabs in order to have their cooperation in minor administrative matters. Lieutenant Wilhelm Langheld, first a member of the *Wissmann-truppe* and later a commander-in-chief of Bukoba, gives an indication of the double task. He listed among his assignments in 1891 the spread of German influence on Lake Victoria, maintenance of contact between the Lake and the coast, and good relations with England. In order to keep his communications between the coast and Lake Victoria open, he did not refrain from punitive expeditions when local tribes or groups of Africans threatened German settlements. On the other hand, he attempted to build up a civilian administration by delegating to native chiefs the administration of their areas and reserved for himself the litigation of disputes arising among the chiefs themselves. As adjudicator of conflicts among the African chiefs he tried to avoid the use of power, at the expense of playing one chief out against the other.[19] Rochus Schmidt reported similarly about his task in Lindi after 1889. The town had been hit hard by the Arab revolt and he admitted that in rising against the new German rulers the people were motivated by justifiable self-interest. He thought he could compensate for past suffering by promoting the economic interests of the Africans, opening up trade between the coast and the interior in the hope that they would overcome their distrust of his administration.[20]

---

[13] Theodor Gunzert, "Die wirtschaftliche Bedeutung der deutschen Kolonien einst und jetzt," p. 106, in: *Kolonialprobleme der Gegenwart* (Berlin, 1939).
[14] Cited in Müller, *op. cit.*, p. 285.
[15] Schmidt, *Araberaufstand*, p. 42.
[16] *Ibid.*, p. 44.

[17] *Ibid.*, p. 258.
[18] R Kol A, no. 745, Bl 95 ff, quoted in Müller, *op. cit.*, p. 552.
[19] Langheld, *Zwanzig Jahre*, pp. 88 and 96.
[20] Schmidt, *Aus Kolonialer Frühzeit*, p. 153.

With the appointment of Freiherr von Soden as the first civilian governor of DOA in 1890 a new phase of civilian central government was inaugurated. Between 1891 and 1901 the second stage of German rule in DOA took shape. It represented on the part of the Africans the transition from active rebellion to resigned endurance of the foreign regime and finally led to cooperation.[21] The new governor set up the departments of justice, public works, health, and agriculture which represented the barest minimum of professional administration.[22] Long-range plans for agricultural and economic development could not be made at this time since indigenous unrest continued in different areas of the Protectorate for a number of years. In 1893 Lieutenant Prince reported from Tabora that for the first time the German prestige could make itself felt, and it seemed that peace was secured although he was aware that resistance was bound to flare up sporadically in a territory as vast as his district.[23] An Arab observer saw it differently in 1892. He described the Africans along the coast as struck with fear of the Germans. It would require special enticements to lure them out of hiding.[24]

An important factor in DOA was the absence of sufficient revenue. Revenue in 1891–1892 was 1,458,000 marks as against expenditures of 3,409,000 marks. By 1895–1896 revenue had quadrupled but the subsidy from the imperial treasury still amounted to 26,111,400 marks.[25] These subsidies continued through the 1890's and affected the expansion of the administration. A definite pattern of government, however, began to emerge. The colony was divided into fourteen districts, each centered on a station governed by a district commissioner (*Bezirksamtmann*). This was a departure from Wissmann's regime although, especially in the beginning, members of the *Schutztruppe* did at times perform civilian administrative services in addition to their military duties. In 1891 the district commissioner replaced the military district chief of the Imperial Commissariat (*Reichskommissariat*). The new district heads were the assessors, men with qualified legal training who lacked, however, the African experience which the *Schutztruppe* lieutenants had acquired in their campaigns into the interior. After 1891 some of the former lieutenants transferred to the civilian administration and added an element of local experience to the group of theoreticians coming from the German law schools. But the problem of coexistence of the civilian and military personnel remained a potential cause of friction. This is borne out by the record of appointments to the governorship between 1890 and 1900. Wissmann's conduct of administrative and financial matters had been criticized by the Foreign Office in Berlin.[26] Freiherr von Soden, Wissmann's successor, performed the duties of governor and central administrator while the command of the *Schutztruppe* was given to a military man, Lieutenant von Zelewski. This arrangement did not prove satisfactory and therefore Friedrich von Schele, Soden's successor, presided over both the civilian and military administrations. In 1895 Wissmann returned to East Africa as governor but the position of commander of the *Schutztruppe* was given to Colonel von Trotha. A year later Eduard von Liebert was appointed governor replacing Wissmann, and again held the governorship and commanded the military forces in East Africa.

These facts make it quite obvious that there were differences of opinion on policy on the part of the Foreign Office in Berlin and the military leaders in DOA. Oskar Karstedt, a former official in DOA whose distorted sense of the German "civilizing" mission in the colony influenced his judgment, may not have been entirely wrong, however, when he attributed the frequent changes of the top personnel in the 1890's to Berlin's lack of understanding of the real needs in DOA. He described the policy of peace at any price as contrary to local needs and described the constant changes of governors as not in the interest of the indigenous population which needed German protection.[27]

By 1901 when Graf von Götzen became governor of DOA and introduced a comprehensive program of colonial development during his five years in office, the political, social, and administrative problems of colonial government had to be taken up systematically for the first time since the arrival of Wissmann's *Schutztruppe* in 1888. It was then, and only then, that serious consideration was given to the operation of government in the colony. Priorities were set up for agricultural production, commercial exports, and industrial exploitation. And behind these issues, and closely interwoven with them, there loomed the all-pervading problems of medicine and public health in a tropical country. The problems were faced at first within the total structure of African colonial government and the solutions devised in the course of the erratic history of DOA present a fascinating though often sad aspect of colonial development.

II. WESTERN MEDICINE AND GERMAN EAST AFRICA: A START

Paragraph one of the decree which established the *Schutztruppe* on February 7, 1889, authorized the spending of two million German marks for "the suppression of the slave trade and the protection of German interests in East Africa." Paragraph two conferred

---

[21] Roland Oliver and Gervaise Mathew, *History of East Africa* (London, 1963), p. 452.

[22] Karstedt described the modest beginnings of the administration, "however modest the administrative organization was—upon its installation the governor had 1 assessor, 1 finance officer, 1 receiver of revenue, 2 bookkeepers and 1 secretary—the problem of finances remained the greatest worry from morning to night." *Der Weisse Kampf*, p. 96.

[23] *Deutsches Kolonialblatt*, 1893. Report by Lieutenant Prince, 29 January, 1893.

[24] Z St A, Potsdam, R Kol A, no 764, Bl 63. Report from Zanzibar by Dr. Carl Reinhardt, 27 March, 1892.

[25] Oliver and Mathew, *op. cit.*, p. 449.

[26] Schmidt, *Araberaufstand*, pp. 300–301.

[27] Karstedt, *Der Weisse Kampf*, p. 100.

executive powers on an imperial commissioner (*Reichskommissar*).[1] The language of the decree was simple; the problems that arose in the wake of its execution were complex. One of the problems stemmed from the difficulties of creating on the spot a competent army with competent officers who would have to be spread over a vast territory which lacked a system of roads. This difficult task was entrusted to Major Hermann von Wissmann.

With the limited manpower at his disposal Wissmann was compelled to distribute his forces over a wide area and created a number of isolated outposts which had to take care of their own needs. The Arabs and Africans, however, who resisted Wissmann's forces had the advantage of being able to move more quickly and change their targets as needed. Ultimately, Wissmann's modern weapons and the support he received from the navy led to the termination of open resistance. But until that happened, his men were exposed to sudden attack and often found themselves without medical help. Several of Wissmann's lieutenants commented on the hidden dangers of those early months.

The *Schutztruppe* started out with two medical officers, chief staff surgeon Dr. Schmelzkopf and staff surgeon Dr. Kohlstock. There were also four medical orderlies.[2] This small number of medical men was inadequate even if Wissmann had been able to keep his forces together. But when small detachments were dispatched to outposts, they were entirely without medical protection. Some of Wissmann's men described the dangers involved. Lieutenant Rochus Schmidt was sent to Mpapua to build up and secure a new station while awaiting the arrival of Stanley's expedition on behalf of Emin Pasha on its way back from Equatorial Africa. His greatest problem was not the threat of attack from African tribes but the outbreak of a devastating epidemic of dysentery. Spread by flies and insects, the epidemic assumed disastrous proportions. "We did not have a doctor," he wrote,

or a sanitary non-commissioned officer. I myself substituted as a medicine man, as many times before, together with Lieutenant von Medem. I must admit that my treatment of dysentery was very poor. My failure to give proper treatment to many white and colored patients burdened my conscience very much. A competent and experienced tropical specialist, and even myself with some training and experience, might have saved many lives.[3]

He was particularly worried about the poor health of his men at a time when his camp at Mpapua was bound to attract worldwide attention after the arrival of Stanley's rescue expedition. How would he be able to conduct his famous protégé safely to the coast in his weakened condition? But the epidemic continued to linger in full force and in his despair he experimented with a most radical medicine recommended by a French missionary. It consisted of fifteen drops of carbolic acid dissolved in a half liter of water. He as well as his men survived and he was able to lead the famous explorers safely "under the German flag through German territory in Africa."

Another man of the Wissmann corps, Major Langheld, told a similar story. He was a commander in Bukoba in 1891. He managed to build up a station surrounded by walls with the help of men who had never been trained as carpenters or masons. But he did not manage to fight disease without the help of trained doctors. He succeeded in administering first aid for injuries varying from wounds to snake bite. But he was unable to cope with internal injuries and epidemics and suffered from a lack of medicine. Yet he carried on and, like the missionaries before him, he recognized that the dispensing of medical help was the best way of gaining the confidence of the African. And this was his goal. He could have done more with even just one trained medical assistant.

The appointment of Dr. Alexander Becker as senior surgeon in 1890 brought considerable improvement.[4] And after the formation of an East African German colonial government in 1891, Becker became the first chief medical officer. Medical officers were now stationed along the coast in Lindi, Pangani, Kilwa, and Tanga but apart from a small government hospital at Bagamoyo, the original base of government operations, there were no facilities for treating Asians and Africans in hospitals. Small facilities at mission stations did not solve the problem of the medical department after 1891. In spite of these limitations the beginning of an embryonic government medical service had been made.

Like its counterpart in the British East African Protectorate, the medical service in DOA was dependent on the limitations imposed on colonial budgets at this time. Administrators in East Africa had realized that plans for the development of the colony must be changed. DOA could not become a reservoir for German immigrants without means. Nor was it as yet ready to harbor a large number of plantations. It was proposed in 1891 to raise the total value of imports and exports above the twenty million mark it had reached between 1889 and 1890. And to achieve this goal, it was argued, Indian capital and the predominantly Indian controlled trade must be replaced by German capital and German industrial output. Then, after the stabilization of the German economy in DOA it would be possible not to depend so heavily on the imperial treasury for the cost of colonial administration. These proposals were presented by Ernst Vohsen, a German administrator in DOA and submitted to the Foreign Office in February, 1891.[5]

---

[1] G. Richelmann, "Wissmann wird Kaiserlicher Reichskommissar," in: *Hermann von Wissmann, Deutschland's grosser Afrikaner,* ed. Richelmann and others (Berlin, 1906), p. 183.

[2] David Clyde, *A History of the Medical Services of Tanganyika,* p. 3.

[3] Rochus Schmidt, *Aus kolonialer Frühzeit,* p. 104.

[4] Clyde, *A History,* p. 4.

[5] D St A, R Kol A 764, Bl 11–12, Denkschrift Ernst Vohsen, DSM, 22 February, 1891.

Dr. Becker, aware of the shortage of funds for colonial expenses, went to a wealthy Indian merchant, Sewa Hadji, to carry out his plan for the construction of a much needed hospital. Sewa Hadji was granted commercial privileges for his commercial enterprises in return for his generosity. He gave to the Imperial Government the sum of 12,400 rupees for the establishment of a hospital and a school which were to bear his name. He stipulated that "the school as well as the hospital were to serve the natives whatever their origin, be they Indians, Arabs, Swahili and the like." The hospital provided for free treatment for the poor. It opened on a limited basis in 1893 with a dispensary, a laboratory, an operating room, and a waiting room. In 1897 it was ready to accept in-patients in its newly built wards for "Askaris, Military Employees and Government Civil Servants." Other patients, according to the official German regulations, such as Indians, Arabs, and Goanese, were also eligible for admission. The hospital served a very useful purpose and was further improved in 1905 by the addition of a new residence hall for its staff. Its admission figures rose steadily.[6] In 1895 the Germans built a government hospital in Dar es Salaam on a healthy spot overlooking the ocean. They further expanded medical stations in the interior where malaria and plague required treatment facilities.

In spite of these improvements a more systematic approach to curative and preventive medicine was not yet undertaken at this time although medical officers were very much concerned about malaria, plague, and the debilitating effects of dysentery. Special projects for malaria and plague control were approved before 1905 but they were not included in the regular annual budgets and were more experimental in nature.[7] As late as 1907 Governor Rechenberg defended government policy toward public health saying that everything was done for the health of the Africans within the limits of the available personnel and the existing funds. He admitted that better public health protection should be introduced in the cities through extended water supplies and better sewer facilities.[8]

But even in the absence of organized research individual doctors were interested in analyzing their observations while they dealt with large masses of the population. From his station in Kilimanjaro, Dr. Brehme, a senior staff surgeon, examined the Wachagga in 1893 and came to the conclusion that there was a relationship between the occurrence of malaria and the altitude of the area. Brehme's successor continued the investigations in 1894. When another doctor systematized his investigations on the relationship between immunity to malaria and its spread in high altitudes eight years later, he had the help of the personnel from the public health service and was supported by the breakthrough in the knowledge of the anopheles mosquito brought about by the experiments of Ross.[9] Plague was explored by Dr. Zupitzer, another medical officer stationed at Lake Victoria. His investigations confirmed its endemic character in the Bukoba district and led to more energetic control. The bacteriologist Dr. Koch consequently organized a campaign to kill rats in affected areas. With these first attempts to investigate serious medical problems, primarily those caused by malaria and plague, the beginning of scientific medicine in DOA had been made. In the succeeding years the services began to grow in volume as can be seen from the annual medical reports. The medical service in DOA started with sixteen doctors and twenty-one non-commissioned sanitation officers in 1895 and reached a total of thirty-six doctors and thirty-nine sanitation officers in 1909–1910.[10]

The unexciting language and the bureaucratic spirit of the official medical reports for DOA do not convey the nature of the dramatic impact which medicine had on the country during the early decades. In the aftermath of the Maji Maji rebellion in 1905–1906 a substantial increase of the staff was requested and granted. Ten new doctors were added whereas it had taken seven years between 1895 and 1902 to get the same increase. The rebellion had made one important point in this respect. It had shown that the social conditions of the African could not be overlooked.

Changes in the organization of the medical services permit further interesting conclusions. The chief medical officer was responsible to the governor who was also commander of the *Schutztruppe* most of the time. But even when the command was unified, the dual task of satisfying the needs of the military and the civilian sector created problems. The colonial medical staff had two categories of personnel, the government doctors (*Regierungsärzte*) and the medical staff officers of the *Schutztruppe*. Government doctors were selected from applications received by the Colonial Office in Berlin. As a rule they must be under thirty-five years of age, unmarried, with clinical experience, and when selected they had to pass a course in tropical medicine at the Hamburg Institute of Tropical Medicine. After appointment they must remain in DOA for a term of at least two years. Their medical duties extended to the European personnel and the indigenous population near their location.

Staff surgeons were recruited from the *Schutztruppe* for which they were primarily responsible. In addition, they were also assigned to the medical care of the officials and the indigenous population. Government surgeons and staff surgeons were given duties and responsibilities which far transcended their numerical

---

[6] D St A, R Kol A 798, Bl 84 and Clyde, *A History*, p. 10.
[7] See chaps. 3 and 4 below.
[8] R Kol A 119, Bl 249, marginal comment by Rechenberg to article on "The Labor Problem," DOA Zeitung, 10 August, 1907.

[9] R Kol A 5838, Bl 4. Dr. Steuber on immunity to malaria, August, 1902.
[10] *Medizinalberichte über die deutschen Schutzgebiete*, 1909–1910.

strength. It was the task of the non-commissioned medical officer to take care of public health and sanitation. They, too, were spread too thinly.

Although a distinction was made between the medical personnel in government and those who belonged to the military, the principal public health officer was not a civilian. He was given autonomy in his department but the execution of policy depended on priorities determined by the governor in DOA and the medical department of the Imperial Colonial Office in Berlin. His recommendations might not carry weight in the light of the governor's program or from the point of view of the Colonial Office. Furthermore, the centralization of the bureaucratic hierarchy of the medical administration required the medical director, as chief medical referee, to report to the medical section of the Colonial Office. This delayed long-range developments although emergencies were taken care of immediately. And it was often because of emergencies caused by malaria, sleeping sickness, and plague that far-reaching policies were developed.

When the shortage of doctors was debated in DOA in 1909, the medical administration came in for strong criticism. Professor Claus Schilling, director of the department for tropical diseases in Berlin, discussed the relationship between staff surgeons of the *Schutztruppe* and civilian surgeons in DOA at a meeting of the German Society for Tropical Medicine in April, 1909.[11] According to his statistics which, he admitted, were not reliable, there was only one doctor for 120,000 Africans assuming that the fifty doctors in DOA were evenly distributed over the seventeen districts. If one compares these figures with those for 1891 when sixteen doctors took care of 5,406,000 Africans, progress was made in nineteen years. The ratio of Africans per doctor had been reduced by one-third while the demand for medical treatment had risen simultaneously. Dr. Schilling deplored the shortage of doctors which could not be justified at the particular stage of development of the colony in 1909. The medical services had been understaffed from the very beginning but there was no excuse for staff shortages after 1905 when fundamental changes in colonial policy had taken place. The country had been opened up. Railroad expansion was planned from Morogoro in the east to Lake Tanganyika in the west. A better-trained staff of civilian officials had begun to provide extended services and new emphasis was placed on public health. What was the reason for the lagging development in medicine?

Back in 1896 Dr. Kohlstock, one of the three doctors who came to East Africa with Wissmann's first expedition in 1889, attributed the problem primarily to the reluctance of doctors to serve as medical staff officers under the prevailing conditions of the service regulations. He found the training of staff surgeons excellent from the medical and scientific point of view. The doctors were well trained to deal with emergencies and new problems of health. But they did not like to serve in the *Schutztruppe* where they suffered from military red tape and had to take orders from regular officers, often of lower rank. Besides, doctors were frequently exposed to greater personal risks without proper protection. Nevertheless he saw advantages in the army discipline accepted by the officers which, in addition to their special training, prepared them to fulfill exceptional tasks as they occurred, for instance, between 1892 and 1894 during the cholera epidemics.[12]

Thirteen years later Dr. Schilling placed more emphasis on the disadvantages of the military-civilian partnership of the East African medical services. He did not find fault with the "excellent work" of the army medical officers whom he found every inch as capable as their civilian colleagues. However, government doctors had the advantage of spontaneity and an open exchange of views. They could freely draw upon the cooperation of the medical profession in the advancement of colonial medicine. They were free to disregard rank in evaluating the fitness and initiative of a doctor. Schilling proposed to increase gradually the civilian sector of the services, especially in the predominantly civilian districts. He assured his audience that he did not advocate an immediate take-over of the military medical services. He found "an energetic military presence of [the German] might in our relations with the natives is still indispensable today in many of our colonies." But he also accused the colonial administrators of not having sufficiently used the doctor as a mediator between black and white in his important task of medical colonization. His critical evaluation of the East African medical services extended further to the powers of the medical director and to the need for more research to be performed in East African institutions.[13]

Schilling was not the only one to be concerned with the need to expand the colonial medical services. Throughout the period one finds in the official correspondence recurring complaints about understaffing and lack of funds and at the same time high praise for the quality of the personnel. If there was a demand for the expansion of the medical department, why did it not occur when it was needed? Was it only a question of insufficient funds? It would be an oversimplification of the complex issues to attribute the problem solely to an "imperialistic colonial" unwillingness to invest money in DOA in the interest of the Africans. It is true that small budgets did not permit the hiring of enough doctors, the building of enough hospitals, and the financing of enough research schemes. But this was only one of the reasons of the existing shortcomings. Preventive

---

[11] Claus Schilling, "Über den ärztlichen Dienst in den deutschen Schutzgebieten," *Archiv für Schiffs-und Tropenhygiene* (1909).

[12] R Kol A 5638, Bl 4–5, Report on the Organization of the German Colonial Medical Services by Dr. Kohlstock, staff medical officer, delegated to Foreign Office, 10 October, 1896.

[13] Schilling, "Über den ärztlichen Dienst," p. 3.

and curative medicine required a better knowledge of the social basis of African life. It could not be undertaken in isolation. It depended on the goals of colonial policy and it changed with the personality of the administrators in the colonial government in Dar es Salaam and in the Colonial Office in Berlin. It was connected with "the labor question" (*die Arbeiterfrage*), one of the central themes of colonial government during the last decade before World War I, but the dependence of "the medical question" on social and political issues was barely understood between 1889 and 1905.[14]

In 1909 Schilling's evaluation of the condition of medicine in DOA pointed in the right direction. He saw the medical services at a disadvantage because they could not respond more quickly to the economic and social growth of the colony. A few administrators had always advocated closer ties with the African population. They saw medicine as an important tool in the pacification of the country because it helped to win the confidence of the people. But policy was made by the top officials and the regular medical officers could not change the direction of the medical services except in their small local realm. As Dr. Schilling saw it, the military organization was not flexible enough in spite of the fact that their civilian counterpart was also restrained, though to a lesser extent, by bureaucratic regulations. Schilling's report was not critical of the significant progress made in the control of the major epidemics of tropical diseases. He was merely concerned with the extension of services in preventive and curative medicine although hospitals had expanded their wards, missions had added trained doctors to their stations, and added treatment had been given to leprosy and mental illness.[15] The time had come to reorganize the services.

This task fell to Baron Albrecht von Rechenberg in 1906. The changeover from military to civilian administration, however, did not become law until 1912 under von Rechenberg's successor Governor Heinrich Schnee. The decree published in the budget of 1912 stated that "in order to have a free hand in the employment of the medical personnel, positions heretofore held by twelve staff surgeons and eighty senior surgeons would from now on be staffed by government doctors" and in order to create a unified budget for the entire medical administration three government doctors were taken over by the department. The budget provided also for the expansion of the medical laboratory in Dar es Salaam into an Institute for the Control of Infectious Diseases and made provisions for the appointment of a civilian medical adviser to the colonial East African government.[16] This change cost the government 116,780 marks. The officials justified these expenses because the Africans had gained more confidence in European institutions through the use of outclinics which had brought them more closely in contact with western medicine.[17] This decree completed the transformation of the medical services from their small beginnings as an adjunct of military government to a full-fledged civilian department in its own right. And it happened just two years before the outbreak of World War I.

The causes of the transformation may be explained in several ways. Official explanations seem to support John Iliffe's thesis that the Maji Maji rebellion initiated major changes in German administration instead of having merely been the reaction to previous actions by the Germans in DOA.[18] Applied to the medical situation, Iliffe's thesis would mean that African action during the rebellion caused the German administrators to react by reorganizing the medical services. In 1906 the Germans admitted that they had overlooked African discontent, and therefore they planned for medical stations throughout the colony as a result of the revolt. But to rely entirely on this interpretation would not do justice to colonial medicine in DOA. As early as 1887 *Schutztruppe* lieutenants had discovered that they could not build up their outposts in the interior without good rapport with the Africans and they noticed that they were more readily accepted as amateur doctors than as builders of military forts.[19] In 1906–1907 and still more in 1912 the advanced stage of colonial development which required the spread of services as well as new policies by the governor and colonial officials led to a more enlightened examination of the role of the African in the German colony. What really happened in the medical services can best be understood by a closer study of the major diseases which had a potential for destruction on a large scale, such as malaria, sleeping sickness, and plague.

III. COLONIAL POLICY AND MALARIA CONTROL IN GERMAN EAST AFRICA

Malaria had threatened the European invaders of Africa from the very beginning. The parasitic character of the epidemic had been demonstrated by Laveran in 1880 but proper and effective methods of treatment were not found until 1900. The apparent hopelessness of the task was expressed in many of the earlier medical reports in German East Africa as well as in the British Protectorate. Staff surgeon Dr. Otto Panse, one of the early participants in the battle against malaria in DOA, described his uneasiness after many years of malaria research in Tanga in a report in 1902 in these words,

the question people ask is whether we dare enter battle in hope of victory or whether, now that we know how danger-

---

[14] See chap. V below.
[15] G. Olpp, "Das Deutsche Institut für ärztliche Mission," *Archiv für Schiffs- und Tropenhygiene* (1909).
[16] TNA, File G3/18, Etat 1912, Beilage 12, pp. 15, 16.
[17] *Ibid.*, p. 94.
[18] John Iliffe, *Tanganyika under German Rule, 1905–1912*.
[19] See p. 10 above.

ous this adversary is, we must despair, not daring to attack but limiting ourselves to mere defense. Should we leave the sword hanging on the wall because it might not be sharp enough, and hide behind the shield, or may we trust in the sword and carry the shield along for as long as we need it?[1]

The sword, in this case, was the frontal attack on the parasite in the blood of affected man with the weapon of quinine, and the shield was prevention through protection against the bite by anopheles and the annihilation of mosquitoes before they could deliver their poison. The results of clinical treatment and the analyses of bacteriologists did not seem encouraging. The number of doctors and researchers in tropical Africa concerned with malaria was not large enough to make a dent into the endless reservoir of the parasites carried by anopheles. The scientists, not generally given to dramatizing their task, sounded emotional when they summarized the results of their work. In the 1890's the habits of the mosquito and the course of the disease were known. The use of quinine seemed to kill the parasite although this was not definitely known until after Dr. Robert Koch made his microbiological analyses in case studies in Dar es Salaam in 1897. But the aetiology of the disease remained a mystery until the Englishman Ronald Ross, an army doctor in India, determined the role that anopheles played in the development of the protozoa which it transferred into the blood of the victim.[2] This breakthrough came in 1898 after four years of intensive experimentation. Until then several alternative approaches to the fight against malaria were explored. One approach attempted to determine whether there were any malaria-free areas which could be reserved for settlement. Another approach evaluated the extent of immunity gained after attacks from which the patients recuperated. There were recommendations to prevent malaria by avoiding "foul air" or by using hygiene. And doubts were expressed that in a country as big as Tanganyika any preventive treatment could be effective. With Ross's discovery of the plasmodium as the amoebic cause of malaria, the choice of alternatives in the struggle seemed to have narrowed down. One must do two things at the same time. One must destroy anopheles near human settlements and one must attack the amoebic protozoa within the blood. Early optimism began soon to give way to further pessimism and forecasts of gloom were frequent. Let us briefly describe the problems of anti-malaria campaigns before 1898. As soon as government had been established in DOA in 1891, fear was expressed that coastal areas would not be safe places for permanent settlement for Europeans. When Drs. Brehme and Widemann investigated malaria near Kilimanjaro in 1893 and 1895, they reported that it was endemic up to 1,500 meters in spite of the apparently favorable mountain climate.

But they found that although malaria existed up to a height of 1,500 meters, it was not as severe as in the lowlands when it did occur, and there were fewer cases.[3] But the outlook even for the highlands of Tanganyika was not bright. There now developed an extended controversy over malaria and the way to fight it. Disagreement basically centered on the following questions. Could the spread of malaria be prevented by medical science and if so, how could the medical profession persuade the government, European settlers, and the vast indigenous population to act according to the recommendations of the experts? One of the very outspoken participants in the debate on malaria was Dr. Friedrich Plehn.

Plehn served as non-military physician in Tanga from 1895 to 1899. In the Cameroons where he had been before coming to Tanga, and later in Tanganyika, he analyzed his findings based on clinical and bacteriological research and questioned the value of the unlimited use of quinine as prophylactic and as therapy. He did not think that quinine must of necessity lead to the eradication of malaria although he admitted that it did help to destroy the residue of the parasite after the attack had subsided. He discussed his findings in 1897 and again in 1901 in articles of the *Archiv für Schiff- und Tropenhygiene*.[4] He saw the problem of malaria as consisting in the choice of selection of priorities. Should emphasis be placed on prevention through hygiene or on the clinical treatment of the malaria patient? Or should an attempt be made to eradicate malaria from tropical colonies to make them fit for white and non-white settlers alike? In 1897 he did not expect results from prevention through sanitation as long as the biology of the protozoa which caused malaria was largely unexplored. His dilemma and his frustration were the result of the tragic isolation in which important discoveries were made as history has shown so abundantly.

While Dr. Plehn saw little hope to find a solution surrounding the "secret" of malaria infection, Ronald Ross was in the third year of his tireless search for the agent of infection by the protozoa. He worked in an isolated army outpost in Bangalore in India. He, too, had been unaware of the many advances in research since Laveran had discovered the movement of amoeboid bodies in the red corpuscles of the blood in 1880. Living under primitive conditions and cut off from the latest biological and medical literature, he made many detours before he was able to describe the growth of the female plasmodium in the gastric wall of the mosquito from where it was transferred to the blood of its human

---

[1] Quoted in David F. Clyde, *History of Medical Services in Tanganyika*, p. 22.

[2] Ann Beck, *A History of the British Medical Services, 1900–1950*, pp. 27 ff.

[3] *Mitteilungen aus den Deutschen Schutzgebieten*, Dr. Widemann, "Bericht über die klimatischen und gesundheitlichen Verhältnisse von Moschi am Kilimanjaro," pp. 296–298.

[4] *Archiv für Schiffs- und Tropenhygiene*, Friedrich Plehn, "Über die praktisch verwertbaren Erfolge der bisherigen ätiologischen Malariaforschung" (1897) and "Über die Assanierung tropischer Malarialänder" (1901).

victim. Ross's patron, Sir Patrick Manson who was medical adviser to the Colonial Office gave his friend advice and much needed confidence during the long months of anxieties and uncertainties when progress seemed to elude him. Ross was haunted by fear and suspicion that premature disclosure of his experiments might steal the victory from under him before he had a chance to present his discovery to the public. Therefore, when the German doctor debated the official malaria program in DOA in 1897, he did not know anything of the most promising approaches to malaria control ready to be proposed one year later.

After Ross's discovery, Plehn still remained doubtful about Koch's method of quininization. Giving full credit to Koch's eminence in modern bacteriology he doubted that the rigid administration of controlled doses of quinine, followed by equally controlled microposcopic blood analyses, would necessarily lead to the disappearance of the disease. What difference did it make to the patient, he thought, to know how many of these little animals he harbored within him as long as this knowledge did not restore him to health? He also criticized the prolonged use of quinine because it influenced the consistency of the blood and he even questioned the ability of quinine to neutralize the toxic substance produced by the parasite. But in spite of these disagreements he consulted Dr. Koch in 1897 to help him with the diagnosis of a "mysterious disease" which he had observed in the Usambara Mountains. This brought Dr. Koch who happened to be in Africa at the time into the twilight area of malaria research on the spot. The mysterious disease was found to be nothing but tertian malaria. Koch had shared the view that malaria occurred only in lowland territory. Now he had to admit that residents of mountainous areas did have malaria.

A new controversy began. The fact that Africans living in altitudes up to 1,500 meters were not spared by malaria caused great concern. What about the healthy "paradise" near Kilimanjaro, dangled before the eyes of would-be settlers? Koch's explanation was that the mountain residents had contracted malaria when visiting in the lowlands and, not having immunity, were more susceptible to more serious cases than their lowland counterparts. But it was shown later that anopheles could live in high altitudes under certain conditions. In 1898 when Koch examined the Usambara mountain area, the issue was not of purely medical concern to scientists. It was charged with political undertones. If the healthy highlands previously described as particularly fit for European settlement were now prognosticated unsafe, then neither the government nor people back home might be willing to invest further in DOA. Neither DOAG nor the planters and the German Colonial Society would allow such negative reports on health conditions in the colony to reach public opinion.

Koch himself permitted his scientific judgment sometimes to be obscured by his conviction that Germany depended on emigration for survival as a great Power. When confronted with East African problems of climate and disease, his answer was that there was disease in Germany as well. "There is no escape from death," he said, why worry? He maintained that the interior of East Africa was healthy and that only the coastal areas should be avoided. He labelled blackwater fever as nothing but a disease of careless quinine takers. And he insisted that since the discovery of quinine prophylaxis, all previous views about the sanitary conditions of East Africa must be thoroughly revised.[5]

For the battle against malaria Koch had developed a plan which stemmed from his preference for microscopic analysis which he considered as the only scientifically acceptable way to deal with a disease caused by a parasite. And the plan for malaria control which he laid down in 1898 when he studied the extent of immunity acquired by different racial groups was based on his experiments with blood slides in his laboratory in Dar es Salaam. He found that smaller doses of quinine were sufficient to cure Africans with semi-immunity acquired over a long period. This would make a large-scale anti-malaria campaign much easier to carry out than a campaign to destroy anopheles over a wide area.

Koch was influenced by his experience on a plantation in New Guinea where 700 plantation workers lived in relative isolation. They were subjected to regular blood analyses under the microscope and treated with quinine as soon as an infection was discovered. After a short time the plantation was free from malaria. This was the scheme which he intended to transplant to Tanganyika where the population moved around freely and the protozoa could also move around freely from one victim to the next and from one place to another. Plehn criticized Koch for ignoring the inability of the doctors to carry out the controlled experiment which, in order to be effective, must reach Africans, Arabs, and Indians alike. In this respect he was right. Another of his conclusions was wrong. He was convinced that the Africans had acquired immunity from childhood on and need not be treated against malaria. He, therefore, came to the startling recommendation to separate African and European living areas, leaving the Africans open to attack by mosquitoes in their unprotected huts while recommending that Europeans be given permanent protection in mosquito-proof houses.[6]

Koch left DOA in 1898 after he had supervised the beginning of a control scheme thought out in the isolation of his laboratory. Plehn's successor in Tanga, the center of malaria investigations, was Dr. Otto Panse who continued the search for immunity from malaria as proposed by Robert Koch. From the examination

---

[5] Z St A, Potsdam, R Kol A 15, Bl 177, 178, Deutsche Tageszeitung, 21 June, 1910.

[6] Plehn, "Über die Assanierung," pp. 45, 48, 49, 51.

of large numbers of blood slides he did not conclude, as did Plehn, that children were immune to malaria but he found that their elders were. Like his predecessors, he sounded alarmed by the slow progress in the battle against malaria and wrote,

the European here with all his modern equipment has the same relationship to malaria that the victorious ruler has to the uncivilized country he has conquered: he is secure in his fortress but dares not leave it, without carrying weapons for fear of being attacked. An East Africa without malaria would resemble a pacified country through which a stranger could pass with only a walking stick in hand. And it is not only the European who would benefit: I disagree with those who claim that the native should be left unprotected from malaria except by immunity.[7]

In 1901 Plehn called malaria "the greatest obstacle of our colonial development."[8] What made it seemingly unconquerable at this time was not so much the medical problem as the question of how to include the African population in the vast scheme of preventive and clinical treatment. In this respect the annual medical reports between 1901 and 1913 are a good indicator of the pessimism of the doctors even though the administrators were careful not to sound too alarmed in order not to affect public opinion at home.

In 1901 Governor Götzen took up the challenge of malaria and asked for special funds from the Foreign Office to begin an organized malaria campaign in Dar es Salaam. Staff surgeon Dr. Heinrich Ollwig, trained in parasitology after he had met Dr. Koch in Dar es Salaam in 1898, combined the latter's method of blood slides and quinine treatment to reduce infection. Meanwhile chief medical officer Dr. Werner Steuber experimented with the elimination of mosquitoes in houses in Kilwa by the introduction of screens. But the experiment was abandoned because the tropical climate led to the destruction of the metal screens in too short a time to make them economical.

Ollwig was helped in his work by a recently appointed health commission in Dar es Salaam[9] which provided technical aid and manpower through the District Office and the Works Department. In addition to inspection of sewers and sanitation, his team examined sections of the population systematically but found it difficult to overcome apathy and antagonism to regular quinine prophylaxis. While it was not easy to deal with a stationary population, it was impossible to subject transient workers to regular examinations. In 1903 Ollwig reported nevertheless that all residents had been examined for malaria every three months in twenty-two districts. In Morogoro and Kilossa he found, however, malaria in 60 per cent of the adults after treatment. Still he continued to share Koch's belief in the effectiveness of quinine as follows from his remark that, "hope for the improvement of these conditions can only be expected if quinine was made available to the natives in large quantities and the carriers of parasites were freed from their parasites in this way." Within limits the malaria control program functioned but the "Expedition for combating malaria in the Protected Territory of German East Africa" was discontinued in 1904. Systematic malaria control was now taken over by the government and the methods of control were broadened. Koch's concentration on the search for the parasites in man's blood was found to be insufficient.

In 1912 the control program among Africans was abandoned entirely when it was found that the number of parasite carriers among children had not been diminished. Dr. Emil Steudel, a former medical adviser to the Imperial Colonial Office, wrote in 1936, "thereby it must be admitted that the systematic program of malaria control according to Koch's plans in Dar es Salaam was abandoned because the hope set into it did not materialize."[10]

Another concern of the doctors in DOA was the damaging effect which malaria had on young children. Here, too, controversial views were developed. In malaria-free territory children were described as healthy looking, exuberant, with full cheeks, whereas in low-lying villages the children had a sickly appearance, were cachectic, and their numbers were small, especially among the Wakami and Waseguna. Blood examinations confirmed the suspicion: the healthy looking children were free from malaria, the others harbored the parasite. These findings made in a report by chief staff surgeon Steuber in 1902 disproved the theory on the naturally acquired immunity after childhood attacks of malaria. He concluded that children either died very early in life from malaria, or if they survived they were not fortified against future attacks later in life.[11] Gone was the fatalism that somehow Africans were better equipped to adjust to the parasite and to fend for their own survival. Dr. Steuber wrote in his 1902 report, "the natives of DOA are therefore, as regards the acquisition of immunity, by no means in an ideal situation."[12]

These revised views on immunity led to a campaign against the mosquito itself and it was carried on in addition to Koch's organized "Expedition" of 1901. The breeding places of mosquitoes in water, household containers, stagnant pools, and in places without drainage were to be eliminated through an all-out effort. The problems which arose with this new approach were staggering. All attempts to educate the people, Africans as well as Europeans, to take quinine regularly had proved to be disappointing. The new approach required Africans and Indians to change their style of life. It also made it very problematic whether the Europeans could be regimented into falling in line with the official request to wage an all-out battle against the breeding

---

[7] Clyde, *History*, p. 22.
[8] Plehn, *ibid.*, p. 41.
[9] Clyde, *History*, pp. 24, 25.

[10] *Deutsch-Ostafrika Gestern und Heute* (1936) Wilhelm Arning, "Koloniale Fragen im Deutschen Reich," p. 192.
[11] Z St A, R Kol A 5838, Bl 4.
[12] *Ibid.*, Bl 8.

places of the mosquito. The campaign was extended to the search for anopheles and continued throughout the German period in DOA.

The official medical reports of the Colonial Office were terse in their description of malaria between 1901 and 1914. Until 1904 malaria took first place in medical reporting when it was directed by the special commission headed by Koch. In 1904, after its transfer to the medical department of the *Schutztruppe* under the senior medical director, it shared attention with many other medical programs in DOA. The changing emphasis in malaria control becomes apparent in the report for 1904–1905. The report pays more attention to climatic conditions, the state of public health in the cities, the living conditions of Africans and Asians. Drainage in Dar es Salaam was taken as seriously as the regular distribution of quinine. But after the revolt of 1905–1906 funds and manpower for the construction of sewers were not available.[13] And as late as 1910 quinine prophylaxis was described as incomplete.

Still another factor entered the picture after the expansion of the railroads. The concentration of railway workers from different tribes, with different customs and ways of living, some of whom had had little contact with Europeans previously, made prevention and cure less promising than imagined by Robert Koch in 1901. When Governor Rechenberg intended in 1910 to close the Kilimanjaro district at least temporarily to German settlers, malaria became a political issue in the debates on settlement in Moshe, Arusha, and Meru, and exposed the governor to attacks by the German Colonial Society.[14] Malaria had not prevented the growth of agriculture and the continued influx of Europeans to DOA but it had created serious delays and obstacles which will be discussed in connection with German social policy in a later chapter.

IV. SLEEPING SICKNESS IN GERMAN EAST AFRICA: SCIENTIFIC EXPERIMENTS AND POLITICAL EXPEDIENCIES

Sleeping sickness occurred in East Africa in 1901 in the British protectorate of Uganda. It was given immediate attention by the Church Missionary Society hospital directed by Dr. Cook in Mengo near Kampala. It alarmed Commissioner Sir James Hayes Sadler and the principal medical officer Dr. A. D. P. Hodges at Jinja on Lake Victoria. Although the British government had in the past dealt with tropical diseases which were epidemic and required strict controls, sleeping sickness added an element of terror and uncertainty and disquieted the small number of officials and doctors who attempted to fight it.

The disease had been known in the Congo before it came to Uganda in the wake of new trade routes with the opening up of Eastern African colonies. It killed mysteriously in its advanced stages and subjected the victims to apathy rendering them unable to lead normal lives. They wasted away very gradually after the nervous center had been affected. Death followed inevitably.[1] The swelling of the glands in the early stages of the disease was soon noticed by doctors and an intensive investigation into the cause of sleeping sickness began. The causative agent, a protozoan called trypanosome, was discovered by Dr. Aldo Castellani in 1903 and confirmed by Sir David Bruce shortly afterwards. This step, however, led only very gradually to a solution of the problem. In the meantime, the disease, though confined to the dense bush and moist climate of Lakes Victoria and Tanganyika, seemed to be terrifying and unpredictable because it did not yield to treatment like malaria, dysentery, and other intestinal infections.

In Uganda sleeping sickness led to the reorganization of colonial administration, it brought about a revision of agricultural and medical policy, and made governors and administrators reconsider their relations with the native population. It prompted the abandonment of fertile agricultural areas under Commissioner, and later Governor, Sir Hesketh Bell in Uganda after 1906 and led to an uproar in the Royal Society in London. It caused disagreement among scholars and scientists in Uganda after the first investigating team had been sent out in 1902. Matters did not become better when the German bacteriologist Dr. Robert Koch came to Uganda to investigate the cause of sleeping sickness in 1903.

By 1906 sleeping sickness had become a scourge which was feared by everyone in Uganda, from the governor down to the men in the bush, although it affected the lives of Africans and Europeans in different ways. Microscopic examinations had shown the presence of trypanosome in the glands and the blood of the patients, and the tsetse fly which throve in the moist vegetation near the lake and the neighboring tropical woods was recognized as the transmitting agent. The process of transmission was not understood until the German doctor Friedrich Kleine proved in 1908 that the fly acted as a vehicle for the development of the protozoa for periods of up to three weeks. Colonial policy in East Africa had been thoroughly put to the test and was not the same again after the shock of 1901 had caused administrative improvisation and led to experimentation in social and economic policies.

Trypanosomiasis came to German East Africa in 1902 when two patients were found afflicted with it in Shirati on Lake Victoria. The cases were thought to have been imported from the British side of the lake in Uganda. Soon after, however, it was discovered that sleeping sickness was endemic on the German side of Lake Victoria, and in succeeding years it appeared in several places. It occurred in the Shirati district and in

---

[13] *Medizinalberichte über die deutschen Schutzgebiete* (1905–1906).

[14] Z St A, R Kol A 16, Bl 13–15, 1911.

[1] See Ann Beck, *A History of the British Medical Administration of East Africa, 1900–1950*, chap. 2.

Bukoba as well as along the coast of Lake Tanganyika. As in Britain, German doctors disagreed on the endemic character of sleeping sickness in their territory, and in one instance, Drs. Feldmann and Lott were reported to have so violently opposed each other that they came close to fighting a duel.[2] Disagreement did not concern the cause of the disease but the method of keeping the tsetse fly out of the reach of human settlements. By 1906 sleeping sickness was considered a serious threat to parts of the shore of the two lakes. On September 26, 1905, Governor Götzen sent an urgent appeal to the Foreign Office in Berlin to speed up the dispatch of an expedition against sleeping sickness and submitted as evidence a report by staff surgeon Feldmann which showed that the disease had spread in the protectorate and that the personnel available for its control was too small.[3] Only two years earlier, in 1903, Feldmann had sounded confident and had minimized the danger of trypanosomiasis. Götzen asked in his dispatch to place Dr. Koch at the head of the expedition to avoid unnecessary conflicts among the experts in the colony. Koch was, therefore, chosen in 1906 when an investigating team was sent to DOA. The problems were not new to Koch. In 1903 when he spent some time in British Uganda, he had visited patients and observed preventive measures taken by the British. He had exchanged views with David Bruce who headed the British sleeping sickness expedition during a very critical period during the initial stages of the epidemic.

Upon arrival in Amani in 1906 where Koch had intended to do research on trypanosome before exploring the affected areas, he received alarming news from Dr. Feldmann about 1,500 to 2,000 deaths in Bukoba the year before, and thereupon left for Mwanza immediately visiting German and British sleeping sickness centers. He was accompanied by Dr. Franz Stuhlmann, a physician and naturalist whose knowledge of the natural habitat of the fly was very helpful. After one month of observations, Koch returned to Germany, leaving Drs. Stuhlmann and Kudicke behind for further research in Amani.[4] Koch confirmed the presence of *G. palpalis* almost everywhere along the coast of Lake Victoria. He was entitled to his judgment since he had proceeded methodically, mapping the incidence of sleeping sickness along the shores of the affected areas. He had collected slides of patients and established camps to isolate them. Among his staff was Dr. Kleine whom Koch selected later as head of a more permanent sleeping sickness control commission. He had failed in his most important objective, to find a cure for the disease and, although he had experimented with atoxyl, an arsenic preparation first used by the British physician Dr. Thomas in Liverpool in 1905, the results of the atoxyl treatment were highly controversial. Atoxyl seemed to arrest the progress of trypanosomiasis if taken early enough but it did not effect a permanent cure and had dangerous side-effects.[5]

In 1907 Koch organized a large and admirable scheme of trypanosomiasis control. His far-reaching plan involved the cooperation of institutions, officials, and a variety of personalities from a wide range of the government, the public health service, the colonial office, the principal medical officer in Dar es Salaam, medical scientists on a large scale, and minor bureaucrats of a number of departments. It was a truly gigantic plan. The aim was nothing less than the eradication of the disease or at least its containment in a limited area in order to preserve DOA as a safe place to live and work. The first meeting of the group was held on November 18, 1907, and the final plans were formalized on December 10, 1907. The expedition got under way early in 1908. No time was wasted and every aspect was considered.

Did the generous planning and the underlying philosophy match the achievements of the commission? Some of the thinking of the policy-makers can best be perceived if one studies the minutes of the session of the subcommittee on sleeping sickness which did the final planning on December 10 in Berlin at the Ministry of Health.[6] During the first part of the session the meeting was presided over by the president of the Ministry of Health while strictly German policy toward East Africa was discussed. The second part of the meeting, concerned with the international aspects of trypanosomiasis control, was chaired by an official of the Foreign Office. Among the participants could be found representatives from universities, members from the department of public health, the colonial office, the German ministry of finance, the principal medical officer of the *Schutztruppe,* and Dr. Kleine, the future director of the control commission. The large number of leading government officials and professional men indicated the paramount significance given to the planning of the operation against trypanosomiasis.

Agreement on the scope of the control commission and its mode of operation was reached after only minor discussion. Dr. Koch had prepared everything well in advance. After his return from East Africa in 1907, he had informed the authorities about conditions in the infected areas and the steps that were needed to be taken immediately. Dr. Steudel, the presiding officer, found his audience receptive toward the plan he outlined. A special appropriation of 809,000 marks was granted. Dr. Kleine was approved as director in control of the entire campaign, appointments to his staff were agreed on without debate. He was allowed six doctors, six public health and sanitation officers, and two sanitation orderlies. He was to have complete

---

[2] Clyde, *History of Medical Services in Tanganyika,* p. 28.
[3] Z St A (*Potsdam*) R Kol A 5895, Bl 92.
[4] *Ibid.,* Bl 99.
[5] Uhlenhut, "Behandlung der Schlafkrankheit," *Verhandlungen des Deutschen Kolonialkongresses* (1910), p. 237.
[6] *TNA* (Dar es Salaam), File G5/16, "Aufzeichnung über die Sitzung des Reichs-Gesundheits-amts," 10 Dezember, 1907.

freedom of action and the right to communicate directly with the governor. Great emphasis was placed on this provision which would give him administrative autonomy within a tightly structured bureaucracy, not an easy proposition for German administrators. It was clear that everyone was aware of the exceptional character of this mission to fight sleeping sickness.

The objectives of the sleeping sickness commission had also been conceived well in advance and did not require discussion at the meeting. In areas affected by tsetse all the inhabitants were to be thoroughly checked for the presence of trypanosome in their bodies. At least four concentration camps for Africans in all stages of the disease were to be erected. Migration across the German-British border was to be prohibited. Examination and observation of the patients, including those outwardly still unaffected but known to be harboring trypanosome, were planned by the medical staff, and research was to be continued indefinitely. It seemed that an operation planned so meticulously must be successful. But officials with experience in East Africa knew that the control commission depended on one important factor which could not be decided upon in the Council chambers. African cooperation must be obtained. Without it neither isolation camps, nor medical examinations, or prescriptions for changes in their ways of living could be enforced, even with the stiffest policing measures. It was agreed to use controls sparingly.

What makes the minutes of the December meeting so interesting is less the outline of a clearly conceived plan to kill and eradicate *Glossina palpalis* and to isolate sleeping sickness victims. Such procedure had been used by the British for several years. More noteworthy is the uncertainty and uneasiness expressed by several of the high-ranking officials, bearers of dignified positions, men used to protocol and rank, when they thought of the implementation of their scheme by those "ordinary" Africans who lived far away and who were the objects of all the planning. Dr. Steudel suggested that, "in order to keep these people in the concentration camps, one must probably resort to gifts and other enticements."[7] The concentrations should be made attractive and the inmates should be treated with generosity. These people must see an advantage in the whole matter, he said, and the men should be permitted to work in their fields and return to their villages during harvest time. One should also think of homesickness, especially among those who were kept in camps without really feeling sick. Strangely enough, Dr. Koch added at this point that he did not expect resistance because the black population was not as sensitive in this respect as "we with our own emotional reactions would make them appear to be."[8] He was entirely wrong in his underestimation of the African sensitivity caused by their strong feeling for home, family, and tradition.

Why did the planners bother to consider popular reaction at all? For one thing, the Germans could spare only a small number of men to control the camps. It would be easy for Africans to escape if they really wanted to do so. The High Command wanted to eradicate, or at least contain, trypanosomiasis, and this required a controlled experiment. And secondly, by 1907 a new trend in colonial policy was under way. After the rebellion of 1905–1906 Governor von Rechenberg, who succeeded von Götzen, and Colonial Secretary Bernhard von Dernburg were determined to promote good will. The methods of Lieutenant von Zelewski in 1888 during the rebellion at Pangani were a matter of the past.[9] The camps were planned for only one year. There was hope that in the meantime better ways of controlling sleeping sickness might be found. The aetiology of the trypanosome was not yet fully known in 1907. The British sleeping sickness expert, Sir David Bruce, assumed that transmission took place directly through the fly from one case to the next. From this theory evolved the policy of limiting the range of the fly. By keeping it within a restricted fly belt after the inhabitants had been evacuated, new infections could not occur in that particular area. Koch, on the other hand, suspected a period of maturation of the protozoa within the fly for several weeks which would necessitate a much more rigid way of separating fly from man. Besides, it was not known in 1907 under what conditions the fly did survive and remain infective. Much depended upon the accuracy with which the various hypotheses about the fly and the trypanosome could be proved. During the planning stage of the control commission there were too many unexplored factors to be certain of the success of any scheme.

In addition to the controversies about control and containment of the fly, there was disagreement on how to treat the patients. Koch believed in the use of atoxyl. It was finally decided to proceed in three major directions at once. First, the forests on Ukerewe Island and near the shore of Lakes Tanganyika and Victoria were to be cleared. Second, four concentration camps were to be erected in which systematic medical examinations were to be given. And third, research into the habits of the fly was to be continued.

Cooperation with Britain was another item on the agenda which required discussion. The British had submitted proposals for an international sleeping sickness bureau. At an international conference earlier during the year in July three proposals had been made. One was the establishment of an international central sleeping sickness bureau to collect data and to take the initiative in international matters related to the disease. In cooperation with the national bureaus of health in each country, the central bureau should have authority to call future conferences. The London proposal em-

---

[7] *Ibid.*, p. 7.
[8] *Ibid.*

[9] Lieutenant von Zelewski, first employed by DOAG and later a lieutenant in the *Schutztruppe* aroused the hostility of the people of Pangani in 1888 by his ruthless enforcement of German rule.

phasized cooperation in the prevention of the spread of trypanosomiasis. The central bureau should be informed of measures taken by the individual countries to enable each member to profit from each other's experience in tropical Africa. A uniform policy of eliminating shrubs and undergrowth near streams and brooks was recommended. The making of maps indicating the geographical distribution of trypanosomiasis was also suggested. All the proposals appeared very useful in order to launch a common attack on sleeping sickness. They stressed practical work as well as research.

A number of German officials and professors were lukewarm toward this proposal. They feared interference with the sovereign rights of the participating states. Dr. Koch found it dangerous to create conditions under which German doctors might be compelled to accept instructions from London. He argued that each country was likely to consider its medical profession superior to that of the other countries and would, therefore, be unwilling to be directed by them.[10] In spite of these and similar arguments, agreement was finally reached that Germany should participate in the proposed London conference in 1908. It was also decided that for political reasons Germany should accept the establishment of an international sleeping sickness bureau on condition that German sovereignty would be safeguarded.[11] There was a strong undercurrent of nationalism in the deliberations which endangered international cooperation by scientists where common interests were at stake.

After his arrival in Dar es Salaam Dr. Kleine took up his task immediately. To establish concentrations for the isolation of the sick, and to keep people in them proved to be more difficult than anticipated. In the district of Bukoba the camps fulfilled their purpose without much trouble. Here the population was under the influence of sultans who consulted with the German representative and influenced the people under their control to accept the German regulations. In the district of Shirati the tribe of the Wagaia, an independent pastoral people, refused confinement to camps. They did not want to be limited in their freedom of movement or subjected to a discipline alien to them. Along the eastern shore of Lake Tanganyika it was even worse. Here the people were less civilized and unable to understand why they should change their style of life. The mere approach of a doctor was the signal for entire villages to disappear. Only the seriously ill were left behind to die which they would have done anyhow. Those still physically and mentally fit enough to move who should have been separated from the rest of the population were left free to spread trypanosomiasis. It also proved very difficult to separate fisherman, laborers, porters, and traders from their accustomed work as long as they did not feel sick. Education was too slow and did not help where superstition, totemism, and native custom were strong and made medical treatment appear as evidence of an evil spirit. In view of the urgency of sleeping sickness control the medical team chose an alternative. They established ambulatory treatment instead of the camps where opposition was strong. Dr. Meixner, principal medical officer in Tanganyika, remarked, "the doctor depends on the good will and compliance by the patient, qualities which are not widely spread among the happy-go-lucky and carefree population."[12] Ambulatory treatment left much to be desired because the patients did not show up regularly.

Dr. Meixner's report leaves out the detail which shows that there were disagreements among the medical sleeping sickness control staff. These show up in the quarterly sleeping sickness reports issued by the Medical Department. In 1909, for instance, it was not easy to recruit laborers for clearing the bush near Lake Tanganyika nor could the personnel be found to erect a camp for concentrations. To enhance the good will of the population, land close to the lake was parceled out and given to those who volunteered to plant food for themselves and the sick, thereby keeping the fly out of the occupied land.[13] In Ujiji Dr. Breuer found an increased number of new trypanosomiasis cases and had to defend the policy of clearing the bush and sanitation. He protested that more cases came to the attention of the authorities because their approach to the indigenous population had been extremely successful. Though by nature very distrustful, the people had lost their shyness because they had become convinced of the peaceful intentions of the doctors and their staff. They brought their sick relatives voluntarily for ambulatory treatment and did not fear to be deprived of their freedom of movement. Dr. Kleine, the director of the Sleeping Sickness Control Commission, endorsed the correctness of Dr. Breuer's report.[14]

In 1912 Dr. Steudel, senior surgeon general, inspected two major sleeping sickness centers on Lakes Victoria and Tanganyika and stated with satisfaction that the original policy of compulsory confinement in camps had been abandoned because it had failed. He described the successful method of clearing tsetse districts even though there was opposition to the seeming waste of manpower and the loss of wooded areas. But he praised the suggestions by Dr. Kudicke who favored the deforestation of large coherent stretches of land near the lake and the abandonment of known tsetse infected land. Since the flying range of tsetse was limited, the cleared area would serve as a protective belt.[15] In his comment on Dr. Steudel's report, Dr. Kleine dis-

---

[10] *TNA*, "Aufzeichnung über die Sitzung," Anlage 2.
[11] *Ibid.*, p. 16.
[12] Hugo F. A. Meixner, "Die Bekämpfung der Schlafkrankheit," p. 261, *Verhandlungen* (1910).
[13] Z St A (Potsdam) R Kol A 5903, Bl 30, 1907.
[14] Z St A, R Kol A, Bl 40.
[15] Reports on sleeping sickness prepared for the German Colonial Office, show that this was one of the principal activities under Dr. Kleine. "Berichte über die Schlafkrankheit in Deutsch-Ostafrika," I, II and III. *Koloniale Rundschau* (1909), pp. 713–749, (1910), pp. 88–112 and 180–189.

agreed completely. He found Kudicke's scheme impracticable because it required more labor than was available for the clearing of the forests. He preferred selective cutting and the limited clearing of areas suspected of *Glossina palpalis* which would serve the same purpose of eliminating the fly, and at the same time, relieve the forest service of the task of destroying entire tracts of bush. As a scientist Kleine was perhaps more skeptical. He cautioned about accepting programs extending over five or more years at a time when medical opinion about sleeping sickness was subject to frequent change. There was as yet too much uncertainty about the period of incubation of the trypanosome in the fly, the potential of a complete cure, and the habits of the fly itself. In 1912 he was not ready to accept a long-range plan which would change the ecology of the soil close to the lakes.

Steudel believed that sufficient progress had been made to contain the fly and the epidemic as soon as a new center of infection was discovered. He was also reassured by the extent of African cooperation in the battle against the disease. Furthermore, he saw sleeping sickness merely as one of many medical problems in tropical East Africa and proposed to be equally vigilant in fighting syphilis and tuberculosis which deserved more serious attention than they were given at the time.[15a]

At the Berlin conference in 1907 Dr. Koch and Dr. Steudel had been optimistic enough to hope that a one-year stay in a sleeping sickness camp would be sufficient and they were confident that sleeping sickness could be eradicated just as cholera and plague had been conquered. In 1912, after years of experimentation, a long and bitter struggle seemed to lie ahead and the outcome was still uncertain when World War I broke out. The colonial government had spent three hundred thousand marks annually on trypanosomiasis control but Dr. Meixner regretted that not all the administrators in East Africa supported the program wholeheartedly.[16] He may have been correct. Colonial Secretary von Solf wrote in 1913 during his trip through DOA, "doctors should not forget, in spite of their preoccupation with sleeping sickness and microscopes, that there are thousands of small ailments which are waiting to be taken care of by the responsible physician, and that a frightening infant mortality requires the treatment of young mothers and their infants."[17] The task seemed endless and the achievements over a period of six years were not decisive. Official recognition was cautious. The doctors themselves, however, saw progress. Dr. Kleine continued his mission until 1914 when he returned to Germany at the beginning of World War I. In an article published in 1941 in *Tropenmedizinische Zeitschrift* he gave a brief retrospective account of his sleeping sickness control mission. He still believed, after all these years, that his mobile treatment centers had served a very useful purpose because they diminished the fear felt by Africans when they were confined in camps. He gave much credit to the policy of eliminating fly-infested woods and their transformation into agricultural land which was then settled with the evicted population. He regretted that the commission's clinical work and its scientific trypanosomiasis research had not led to final results when war broke out in 1914.

As for the British continuation of sleeping sickness control in Tanganyika, he gave them credit for their work but he criticized them for having failed to recognize the threat posed by *Glossina morsitans* which transmitted sleeping sickness to humans in addition to *Glossina palpalis*.[18] He blamed them for not having continued his policy of resettlement although the British had developed the policy of abandoning land to the fly when the population was sparse and of resettling it on a large scale when the population was dense. Between 1905 and 1927 they had been very flexible in making their policies dependent upon economic and demographic conditions.[19] Kleine concluded his article with an outline of a German program of sleeping sickness control which he expected to introduce after the end of World War II assuming that the Germans would reestablish their control over the former colony.

Comparing the German and British policies toward sleeping sickness significant differences become apparent. The British had in 1901 stumbled into a situation for which they were not prepared. Unable to stem the outbreak of sleeping sickness in Uganda, they resorted to untested remedies. Between 1901 and 1903 the sick were taken care of in emergency wards to relieve their suffering which always ended in death. The officials were terrified by their inability to help. Doctors in Uganda and in England were unable to come up with answers. An atmosphere of gloom prevailed in 1903 when government officials witnessed the personal rivalries among members of the first scientific team reaching Uganda from London. Their confidence, however, was restored when Sir David Bruce confirmed Castellani's identification of the trypanosome as the cause of sleeping sickness in 1903. It was now possible to devise a strategy for attack, and a succession of governors and principal medical officers carried out the withdrawal of the population from Lake Victoria until they recognized that economic and social considerations were as essential in sleeping sickness strategy as purely curative measures and research. They experimented with wholesale transfers of the population from unsafe villages and placed the involuntary migrants into new settlements

---

[15a] Z Sta A (Potsdam). R Kol A, Bl 78.
[16] Meixner, "Bekämpfung der Schlafkrankheit," p. 270.
[17] Bundesarchiv (Bonn), Nachlass Solf/36, "Diary of a trip through Africa, October 4, 1913, p. 32.

[18] Friedrich K. Kleine, "Die Schlafkrankheitsbekämpfung in Ostafrika vor und nach dem Kriege," *Deutsche Tropenmedizinische Zeitschrift* (1941), pp. 28, 29.
[19] Ann Beck, *A History of the British Medical Administration*, pp. 114–126.

where they had an opportunity to improve their standard of living. They saw to it that they learned better agricultural techniques which would enable them to have a better life. Often they failed, in part because Africans refused to give up their customary way of life or because of homesickness for their old places and out of fear to accept change. But whether officials failed or succeeded, they were passionately involved in what they did.[20]

The British sleeping sickness program was not as centrally administered as that of the Germans. In London it depended on decisions by the Colonial Office, the Royal Society, and the School of Tropical Medicine. In Uganda a number of administrative agencies, such as the Department of Agriculture, Native Affairs, Entymology, and the Department of Medical Services contributed more independently than in DOA. Action might be delayed because of departmental disagreements or because a new governor arrived and reversed his predecessor's strategy or because the entomologist disagreed with the forestry department. But in spite of controversies and delays the program was successful and its history shows an awareness of the social and economic implications of trypanosomiasis in relation to African society.

The German program was carried out according to the original master plan conceived by Koch and amended by Kleine. When Kleine translated the blueprint into action on the soil of East Africa, he and his medical staff became aware of the need to gain the support of the Africans which forced them to make their program more flexible than originally anticipated. Throughout the years of German control of sleeping sickness in their East African colony, the program remained efficient and reflected the stamp of officialdom.

V. SOCIAL POLICY IN GERMAN EAST AFRICA: PUBLIC HEALTH, MEDICINE, AND THE LABOR QUESTION

Labor policy in German East Africa underwent considerable changes under consecutive colonial governments.[1] Most of the changes occurred as the goals for export crops and commercial development were revised in the light of more favorable living conditions and the improvement of health. In the early days labor was primarily seen in terms of porters for expeditions and commercial enterprises. After the colonial government thought of attracting European settlers for plantations and industrial establishments, the recruitment of labor became a key factor in colonial policy. Since colonies received only minor subsidies for their operational budgets in the 1890's, and were even expected to become self-supporting in the not too distant future, economic development seemed to be a necessity in the interest of the colonial government.

During the first decade after the establishment of the protectorate, farms and plantations did not progress as expected because of insect pests, lack of roads, and lack of manpower. This happened in British East Africa, too, where the initial failure of Lord Delamere's attempts to breed cattle would have discouraged the less determined and less affluent settlers who could not absorb the losses. In German East Africa larger plantations developed only slowly before 1903, and although workers were needed on a smaller scale, the problem of labor (*die Arbeiterfrage*) began to arise even then, and became a standard item in the major colonial publication *Deutsche Kolonialzeitung* for the remainder of the period. It was also frequently commented upon in the official correspondence between the Colonial Office in Berlin and the governor's office in Dar es Salaam.[2] Many of the proposals of how to channel African labor into farm work, road construction, and mining enterprises varied from utter naïveté to sophisticated suggestions based on economic and social theories on the nature of colonial labor.

In general British and German estimates of potential improvements in the quality and quantity of African labor were pessimistic. Sir Charles Eliot, the first British commissioner of the East African Protectorate, decided to introduce a hut tax in 1902, but not as a device of increasing the work force. He thought merely of getting revenue in order to appease his critics at home who begrudged the subsidies that were paid for the colonies. Besides, Eliot did not think highly of Bantu labor in Kenya and their ability to produce more than a subsistence economy. Comparing them to the gifted Baganda in Uganda, he considered the Africans in Kenya as unqualified to create a civilization since they were "somewhat low in the scale of civilization and had no political organization."[3] They live, he wrote, "in a country exposed to sudden natural visitations, but are not sufficiently civilized to prevent or in any way mitigate floods, epidemics or drouths," their chief idea of activity being the waging of wars.[4] Toward the end of his term, however, he concluded that "the natives [had] of late shown a docility and aptitude which was hardly anticipated, and had proved that they can and will work not only in the fields but at various mechanical crafts in the railway workshops."[5] Eliot considered the question of African labor within the context of the development of Kenya for European trade and the settlement of European farmers. Within this framework, he was ready to concede to the African

---

[20] *Ibid.*

[1] This chapter is limited in scope. Even so, it seems to transgress the subject matter of the book. In assessing the role that medicine and working conditions played in relation to living conditions and human improvement in DOA, a discourse on the theory of colonialism has not been attempted. For a more recent study of this theme, see Rainer Tetzlaff, *Koloniale Entwickelung und Ausbeutung* (Berlin, 1970).

[2] Z St A (Potsdam), R Kol A vols. 118–124.
[3] G. H. Mungeam, *British Rule in Kenya, 1895–1912*, p. 109.
[4] Sir Charles Eliot, *The East Africa Protectorate*, p. 98.
[5] *Ibid.*, p. 173.

a role in the productive economy commensurate with his natural gifts as reflected in his past achievements.

In German East Africa, too, the problem of getting a modest revenue from their colony and the difficulties of obtaining a satisfactory labor force for an expanding economy were recognized from the outset. In 1898 a hut tax was introduced with the comment that the Africans should contribute to the revenue in return for services they received, such as protection and better roads. It was not linked to the recruitment of labor. In fact, the recruitment of labor did not become acute at that time. Labor shortages did not become critical until after the government entered into competition with private business under Governor Götzen.

Until World War I the "labor question" was part of a wider problem, also identified as the "social question" or the "African question." It became a grave issue when European planters as well as government projects faced a shortage of labor. When in such emergencies they suddenly noticed that African peasants resisted plans to transfer them in larger numbers to places of work which were far away from their villages, they began to wonder why their relations with the indigenous population were not what they ought to be. In 1893 DOAG opposed Governor Schele who issued a decree which was interpreted as too friendly toward the African because it proposed to educate him and train him for work on plantations.[6] By this time it was recognized that agricultural development on the plantations could not progress unless a sufficient reservoir of labor could be utilized at any time. An earlier experiment in 1891 to import some hundred laborers from China and Japan had been a failure. After that, one had tried to recruit the Wanyamwesi who were induced to settle near Pangani in 1895 but the result was equally disappointing.[7] When more plantations began to operate by the end of the century, German settlers became impatient and demanded that they be given priority on the labor market. At the same time the German government began to insist on regulations in the interest of a long-range labor policy. Such a policy, in addition to procuring the physical bodies needed for work, should also improve the quality of labor and adjust African living conditions to what the Germans expected African villages to be in the future.

With the arrival of Governor von Götzen in 1901 more far-reaching projects of resettlement for Africans were attempted. District Commissioner Ludwig Meyer proposed in 1901 to settle the Nyamwezi in the Usambara mountains close to European plantations where they would serve as a reservoir of labor and produce marketable crops near the coast. Götzen also contemplated a scheme to develop in the African an interest in local communities (communes) by a decree in 1901 which, on paper, had a progressive flavor.[8] Income collected in the communes would not only relieve the official budget by financing local expenditure through local taxes but it would also help to "educate" the African. Responsibility given local people in the communes would strengthen their personality by giving them a voice in their own affairs. At it turned out, however, the communal organizations shared their income with the military districts by up to 10 per cent to compensate them for services and payments to jumbes. African representation in the district council, originally decreed in 1901, was abandoned in 1903 because, as Götzen explained, the experiment had failed during a trial period of three years. He was disappointed, he wrote to the Foreign Office, that local participation had not served to educate the African along the lines of German virtues thereby helping to spread German prestige. He insisted that the most intelligent Africans had been given an opportunity to participate in meetings of the District Council but they had been unable to participate in the deliberations because they failed to understand the discussions. He also mentioned that Europeans on the Council did not want to air their problems in the presence of Africans. As a way out of the dilemma Götzen proposed to make the knowledge of the German language a prerequisite for nomination to the Council, a device which he knew would *de facto* eliminate African representation for the next twenty years.[9]

Although Götzen hoped to increase the African contribution to DOA's agricultural economy, his scheme of increasing peasant output by introducing them to the growing of cash crops was a failure because it was poorly conceived. The idea in itself had merit, but having neglected to establish an understanding between the official advisers and the village producers, Africans in the Southern Highlands did not trust the motives of the German plan. Forced to plant sisal, rubber, and coffee instead of copra and peanuts, without having been prepared for the new undertaking by education, they resisted the change in their lives and were determind to return to their tribal tradition. The result was a violent reaction which manifested itself in the Maji Maji revolt in 1906.[10]

In the meantime the expansion of the agricultural economy of the planters made them more insistent than ever to demand their right to recruit labor by any means, even if it meant outright compulsion. They resented government regulations by the colonial administrators and denounced them as unwarranted interference in their lives. On the other hand, quite illogically, they felt that they were entitled to active government support in the recruitment of labor and presented themselves as engaged in a fierce struggle for survival in the face of the harsh realities of the tropical climate and its diseases. Over the years the attitude of the

---

[6] Z Sta A, R Kol A, Bl 3.
[7] H. Brode, *British and German East Africa*, p. 87.
[8] Z Sta A, R Kol A 798.
[9] *Ibid.*, Bl 188/189, 1903.
[10] Kenneth Ingham, *History of East Africa*, p. 197, and John Iliffe, *Tanganyika under German Rule*, p. 23.

planters had stiffened considerably. In 1893 DOAG had reproached the Foreign Office for its interference in its private rights. They had asked how the imperial government dared to burden them with regulations on labor at a time when they were the pioneers in a colonial economy still in its embryonic stage. Why did Governor Schele not understand, they queried, how damaging these government regulations would be for economic development in East Africa?[11] In 1894 *Hamburger Nachrichten* echoed the same point and attacked Schele's views as erroneous because he proposed some training for Africans to make them more useful on plantations. From the planters' point of view the labor problem involved only the organization of a steady flow of workers to all centers of employment.[12] The debate on labor remained substantially unchanged between 1890 and 1900. The settlers did not examine the underlying causes of the labor shortage nor could they do so as long as their attitude toward the African remained unchanged. They insisted that he was obligated to work and that government was "much too timid and concerned with the psychical balance of our natives."[13] The German Colonial Society described the Negro as shiftless and disapproved of his tendency to move about the country (*Wanderlust*) because these qualities made him a very unreliable worker. The Society demanded that the government not hire these runaway workers and issue regulations which would aid the settler in his desperate struggle for survival.[14] St. Paul Illaire, director of the East Africa Company, attributed the problem of labor less to a dissatisfaction with wages than to a difference of life styles. "Many tribes," he wrote, "adjust their work to their convenience; they hoe a small piece of land today, and another one tomorrow; no one drives them. If it rains, they go into a hiding place, and, if the sun is too hot, they look for shade. What they cannot finish today, can just as well be done tomorrow. The absence of any discipline, any kind of control, characterizes this kind of working habits [on their own fields]."[15] Working, however, on European plantations where expensive and seasonable crops must be taken care of intensively and without interruption, the African might conform to the new demands and "even" be called industrious. But he also might rebel and refuse to change his ways, especially when not knowing why he should do so. The planter who took it for granted that labor in the colony must serve his class regardless of the preexisting cultural pattern of the peasants, became more dogmatic and passionate as he was fighting on two fronts. He condemned the colonial administration as well as the natives whom he had failed to control.

Under Götzen's regime, an open break was avoided. But Götzen's plan for a diversified agricultural economy did not materialize.

The labor situation did not immediately improve under Governor von Rechenberg. From a purely statistical point of view, there was no reason to despair. With a total population estimated at four million and only 23,000 needed for the labor force in 1905, the number of men working at the time was 13,000. It was, therefore, a political problem to get the full contingent of labor which the planters claimed to be essential for their economic survival. It depended on them and their choice of a social policy. The new men concerned with colonial policy were Bernhard Dernburg, Germany's first colonial secretary, and Governor von Rechenberg, the successor of Götzen. They recognized the political aspect of the "labor question" and therefore changed their approach to the problem accordingly.

Rechenberg sought to improve the process of recruitment and searched for new standards in the treatment of African labor. Before his time freewheelers had collected African laborers indiscriminately, sending them to the highest bidder without telling them what was expected of them. The speculative recruiters went from one plantation to the next, concerned with the highest offer from the planters, and then sent the men to those who paid the highest commission. The potential workers were not matched with their jobs. The planters themselves were not satisfied with these methods and formed a syndicate in 1905 to share the expenses and have better recruiters. They selected a Mr. Tomaschek who would receive a fixed salary based on the immediate partial payment of the syndicate's capital pledged by the ten largest plantations. When the planters did not live up to their pledges, Mr. Tomaschek reneged on his agreement and the old methods continued.

Rechenberg tried to institutionalize the recruitment of labor within the colonial administration which had been reorganized after the revolt of 1905. Both Dernburg and Rechenberg were determined to get at the root of the lag in productivity in DOA and the reasons for the lingering resistance by the planters. They also wanted to know why the majority of African peasants were accused of apathy in their dealings with planters, settlers, and other employers. Most of the complaints about the quality of African labor seemed to attribute its failings to lethargy and apathy.

One of the first things Rechenberg did was to recommend a labor recruitment company (*Arbeiteranwerbegesellschaft*), to replace the abortive privately promoted syndicate of 1905. At a meeting of the German-East African plantation society in Berlin in 1907 Rechenberg announced as his priority a better system of worker recruitment. The colony was bound to lose money and its credit at home unless it was able to produce a cooperative labor force in the colony, he

---

[11] Z Sta A, R Kol A, 118, Bl 8.
[12] Z Sta A, R Kol A 118, Bl 20.
[13] *Ibid.,* R Kol A, 119, Bl 48.
[14] *Ibid.,* R Kol A 118, Bl 98.
[15] St. Paul Illaire, "Die Arbeiterfrage in DOA," *Deutsche Kolonialzeitung* 25 (1908): p. 19.

argued. He criticized the abuses known to have happened in recruitment, especially in the interior of the country. If the planters complained about wages of fifteen rupees being too high as compared with wages of eight rupees paid by the railway companies, they forgot that railway workers received food, living quarters, and medical care in addition. "If I say," the governor continued, "that we shall attempt to regulate this matter, we want to stress the fact that the procurement of workers is the most important thing. If we concern ourselves with labor recruitment, we are interested in protecting the reputation of the plantations threatened by the excesses of the recruiters."[16] In spite of this strong language and repeated exhortations by the governor, the labor recruitment company was not set up until March 11, 1909. In October of the same year the debate on whether the company which existed on paper should become active and really recruit workers had become acrimonious and exasperating, like previous discussions on labor ever since Rechenberg's arrival in 1906. The organization of German East African planters demanded a government subsidy to match the high wages of fifteen rupees. In 1910 planters and governor were farther apart than they had been in 1906 because they disagreed radically on what constituted "decent working conditions." Rechenberg hoped for economic improvements in the colony and warned plantation owners saying "gentlemen, economic growth and falling wages, that cannot be done, neither here nor in the colonies,"[17] while the planters responded with a refusal to invest any more money in the labor recruitment scheme and continued to insist that wages must be kept down.[18] Even in 1911 the society for the recruitment of labor did not function in spite of a decree of 1909 which had placed the recruiter firmly under the colonial administration and had set guidelines for labor contracts limiting their duration to seven months or 180 working days so that Africans would not be separated from their families for indefinite periods.[19] It also gave the worker at least nominal legal representation by appointing the district commissioner as his legal representative. It is clear that the two sides were unwilling to arrive at a mutually acceptable policy on African labor. It is also clear that the main ingredient for cooperation was missing because confidence in the governor and his colonial secretary had been successfully undermined by a continuous series of attacks on them in the influential *Usambara Post* and *Koloniale Zeitung*. This is not the place to analyze Rechenberg's and Dernburg's colonial policy. But a brief explanation of their views is necessary to grasp fully the incongruity of the situation.

In 1907 Secretary Dernburg exposed his views frankly in a letter to a German employed in a mining enterprise in DOA. Apparently he expected that his views would be made known because he added this sentence to the letter, "If you should desire to make use of my communication, you need not hesitate to vouch for its authenticity."[20] The writer had asked for Dernburg's opinion in his anxiety about the steadily deteriorating relations between officials and non-officials in DOA. Dernburg referred to the uniqueness of conditions in the colony which compelled the colonial government to exercise pressure in two directions, on workers as well as on settlers, in order to restore a minimum of cooperation. Because of this uniqueness, the government must exercise pressure on African peasants to induce them to work for the settlers. In doing so, however, it must also assume responsibility for their treatment. In many proven cases working conditions were very bad and it was understandable that under these circumstances, "the blacks did not like to work for certain whites and that, on the other hand, the district officers hesitated to make the black men work for them." But the labor problem was more than the problem of the native in his relationship to the European. Much more important, perhaps, was the entire problem of colonial development and its dependence on native production. He was convinced that the economy of East Africa could not depend on the operation of some fifty to sixty plantations and settlers but that it must develop in conformance with its natural products, its native production, the natural experience of its native population and that, with all due care for the European capital invested in the colony, the development of the native economy was the safest way to relieve the German state of its payment of subsidies and to open the way for a broad colonial policy.[21] One has here a good example of "enlightened colonialism" which placed emphasis on Germany's economic needs and stressed consideration of German colonial budgets. But once this premise was accepted, the treatment and welfare of the African were taken seriously and remained the undisputable concern of the state.

On the other hand, colonial spokesmen for plantation owners rejected Dernburg's assumptions. W. von St. Paul Illaire, a director of the East Africa Company, wrote in *Deutsche Kolonialzeitung* in 1909 about the large numbers of Germans who distrusted the intentions of the colonial government. He saw merit in Dernburg's plan to have a labor commissioner responsible for labor recruitment which should be done with a minimum of friction and anxiety among the Africans. But he doubted that such a plan could succeed without having reached a prior agreement between government and settlers on how the native question was to be solved. Illaire took a very dim view of the implementation of Dernburg's policy.

---

[16] Z St A, R Kol A 120, Bl 15, 20 December, 1907.
[17] Z St A, R Kol A 120, Bl 51.
[18] Z St A, R Kol A 528, Bl 27.
[19] Z St A, R Kol A 528, Bl 33, 1911.

[20] Z St A, R Kol A 120, Bl 16.
[21] Z St A, R Kol A 120, Bl 15.

A much more outspoken criticism came from the northern branch of the German Economic Association in 1907. In a memorandum to the Reichstag they informed the German Parliament of the radical differences of views held by the colonial administration on the one hand, and most of the Europeans in the colony on the other hand. Remarks by Dernburg indicated that, "in DOA a native policy was to be pursued which favored exclusively the interests of the black population, neglecting German economic interests, i.e., a policy designed to make DOA exclusively a Negro- and Indian-commercial colony." The secretary of state and the governor did not even admit that a labor problem indeed existed in the colony. This, they maintained, was entirely wrong.[22] What they did not admit was that they were unwilling to accept the Dernburg-Rechenberg plan to solve the labor problem by applying pressure as well as good will to affect a change in the direction of a colonial social policy, giving more flexibility to African agriculture, even at the expense of the pool of manpower available for German plantations.

Dr. Arning, a medical officer during the pioneer period of colonization and a member of the Reichstag in 1908, discussed the "native question" at a board meeting of the German Colonial Society in a more enlightened way. He rejected the notion that the Negro was incapable of doing work in the European sense. He found individual differences in their abilities, just as they existed between a North German hard-working peat-cutting peasant and the Italian loafer in the south of Europe given to *dolce far niente*. He found exaggerations about the African's ability or inability to work not conducive to the solution of the problem of labor. Neither the legend of the lazy African nor the lavish praise by political liberals like Dernburg could lead to a solution of the problem. Neither view was correct since it overlooked the disparity of living conditions in Africa and Europe.

Dr. Wilhelm Solf, colonial secretary from 1911 to 1918, visited East Africa in 1912 and came to conclusions very similar to those of Dernburg. Unlike Dernburg, who was unable to penetrate below the surface of African life during his hurried visit in 1907, Solf took time out to meet planters, and listened to their criticism of government regulations of labor recruitment. He undertook long trips on the recently constructed rail links to the interior and met with engineers and technicians. He talked with government officials in Lindi, Dar es Salaam, Morogoro, and Tabora, and on occasions mixed with Africans in the manner of a campaigning politician. He came to the conclusion that the German colony was not a white man's country. Its future prosperity depended on enterprises with a minimum investment of 30,000 marks. He did not see a future for medium-sized European farm holdings. African peasant holdings on the other hand seemed to him essential as did a labor force capable of improving its quality and its standards. His impressions of African villages were favorable. He wrote,

We came for hours past villages which were kept very clean. Also the herds of cattle made a very good impression. Little remains of the image of the lazy Negro described by the planters and envisaged by the public at home, if one has seen the fields of the natives around Tabora.... He who sees the Negro solely as *corpus vile* for his own economic purposes, should stay at home. In the colony such people only disturb the quiet progress and damage the reputation of the colonies through their noisy propagation of false views in the press at home.[23]

When he visited railway construction projects, he found their quality comparable to similar work done in Europe by European labor. In talks to delegates of the East African Economic Association who had come to complain about conditions in the colony, he said that it was not the government's fault that a labor question existed. This, he reminded them, was an issue common to all white settlers in all African colonies. "While the planters approached the labor question solely from the perspective of its limited application to the interest of the white planters," he argued,

they ought to recognize that seven million natives were not a *quantité négligeable* to the government. The government could not do anything else but draw the proper diagonal in the parallelogram of conflicting interests. If they did not like the diagonal, they could not complain about a lack of interest by the government but should attribute it to the endeavor to do justice to both sides.[24]

Toward the end of the trip the colonial secretary wrote in his diary that he had confidence in Governor Schnee's ability to work out a policy for East Africa which would harmonize the interests of the Europeans with those of the Africans.[25] There is no doubt that Solf was sincere in his favorable judgment on East Africa's potential for development. He did not minimize the uncooperative attitude of the settlers but refused to be discouraged by a phenomenon which he dismissed as a temporary inconvenience. He believed that it was possible to have a peaceful and productive colony sooner or later supported by the diligence and ability of seven million Africans protected by the German government.

In spite of Solf's utopian vision, settler opposition to German labor policies remained unchanged to the end of the colonial period. A memorandum presented by the Economic Association of Kilimanjaro to Secretary Solf and Governor Schnee during their visit to the area in 1912 does not differ much from similar memoranda written in 1907. Members of the Association expressed their preference for a system of cards which would oblige every adult man to work a minimum of ten days for one employer each month in order to compensate the government for the expenses

---
[22] Z St A, R Kol A 120, Bl 89 and 91.
[23] Nachlass Solf, 136, Bl 65/66.
[24] *Ibid.*, Bl 62.
[25] *Ibid.*, Bl 79.

incurred in support of the colony. In their opinion colonial subsidies by the German Treasury helped primarily the African population and, therefore, the Europeans were entitled to a bountiful supply of labor in return. They insisted that progress depended on labor and, since the Africans were not yet able to understand why progress was in their own interest, it was the "duty of the colonizing nation, in the interest of the education of the Negro, to use the power of taxation in order to create conditions which would guarantee the cultural progress of the country."[26] And so it happened that the German government found itself in the role of protector of African labor. Ironically, this role assumed ever larger proportions with the expansion of the network of railroads, the increased investment by industrial companies, and larger exports of raw materials. Official concern with the health of African workers, whether in government service or in private plantations, became a necessity. It is interesting that research in botany and agriculture began as early as 1902 whereas scientific medical concern with the health of the men who produced the harvests and built the roads, railways, and ports did not begin until the Rechenberg administration.

The activities of the Philip Holzmann Company offer a good example of these changing attitudes. The company was among the major builders in DOA. The railroad it built in 1911–1912 was to run from Morogoro to Tabora and led through sleeping sickness-infested territory. Excavations created uneven earth levels in which stagnant rain water accumulated as soon as erosion set in, thus creating ideal breeding places for malaria mosquitoes.

Large numbers of laborers passed through these areas during construction. It was here that the commissioner of railways averted serious danger through inspections and regulation. He sent reports to the governor, the medical department, and other officials, and alerted them to health hazards from sleeping sickness. The relationship between the railway commissioner and the private companies was not always too cordial between 1910 and 1915. The government wished to maintain a uniform policy on all railway projects and programs of deforestation which often preceded the extension of the railways.[27] In tsetse-infested territory this was very important and included some supervision over the hiring of labor, and its proper housing, feeding, and medical treatment. The railway commissioner, as the annual report stated in 1910, was the official representative of the government and as such he was responsible for the regulations relating to the construction of railways. The reports which the commissioner sent to Governor Schnee during the building of the Tabora-Kigoma line give regular accounts of inspections of the workers' camps and their health by a government-appointed doctor. They also show that the commissioner's directives were often disregarded. The private companies which operated without government subsidies balked at suggestions of costly measures of preventive sanitation which were not stipulated in their contracts. The Holzmann Company, one of the largest, operated under a contract which specified the government's right to supervise the progress as well as the quality of works.[28] But the company tried to avoid compliance when government supervision became too demanding. In a letter to the governor, manager Hoffmann of the Holzmann company strongly objected to the accusations of bad treatment of his workers and denied irregularities in management or unwarranted dismissal of workers. He put it simply to the governor, writing, "Your Excellency will find it understandable that it is impossible to respond to the wishes of every single man in an enterprise as vast as ours." He assured him that as far as possible due consideration was given to the different habits of the various tribes while special efforts were made to maintain regular payment schedules and good treatment.[29] If the commissioner wanted to see the railway nearing completion as fast as possible, he could not make full use of his legal powers to enforce regulations. The workers, on the other hand, did seem to prefer employment with large construction companies to work on plantations. Although at first averse to regular health checkups which construction workers were forced to undergo, they gradually began to appreciate medical care when they felt the benefits they derived. They appeared voluntarily at native hospitals in neighboring towns. Statistics indicated a decline of the death rate due to accidents, suicides, epidemics, and overwork. The death rate for 20,000 railway workers was down to 141 in 1912 from 422 in 1909.[30] In 1913–1914 the death rate for all construction workers was only 2.3 per cent of the work force.[31]

But health was not the only item singled out by the railway commissioner in his report. He concluded that the general condition of labor was better than in previous years. There were many among the workers who were willing to accept contracts for as long as six years, a fact which he interpreted as an expression of satisfaction with their work. He was also satisfied to note that recruitment did not present a problem any more for government-sponsored employment. But there remained another matter of great concern. As the railway approached Lake Tanganyika, it could cause the dispersal of the testse fly from its habitat in the dense bush from where it might then threaten a new area which up to this time was free from trypanosomiasis. This risk must be faced squarely as the lesser of two evils. It was preferable to the grave disadvantages

---

[26] Memorandum by Economic Association of Kilimanjaro to Secretary of State Solf, Nachlass Solf, 33, Bl 252/253.
[27] TNA, G12/208, Bl 59.
[28] Ibid., Bl 109/110.
[29] Ibid., G12/165, Bl 1/3, 1911.
[30] Ibid., G 12/5 Bl 29, 1912.
[31] Ibid., G12/16, 1913–1914.

of porter traffic carried on for so many years. Infected porters who were not aware of their condition had for many years carried trypanosomiasis from the unsafe shores of Lake Tanganyika to the coast which was generally free from infection. By the abandonment of porter traffic and by the creation of a modern system of transportation trypanosomiasis could be controlled and the porters could be rehabilitated under socially improved conditions. The Wanyamwezi who contributed so much to porter traffic could then again lead a stationary life, preserve their culture, and "stem the physical and moral decay of a tribe which must be counted among the culturally most advanced tribes of Africa." [32] The moralizing and patronizing tone of the railway commissioner's analyses contrasted with the pragmatic evaluations of the men who actually directed the operations. The manager of the Holzmann Company, his engineers, and his technicians pursued their difficult and not so romantic task of linking west central Tanganyika with the modern world. They did not describe themselves as heroes of a cultural mission but they expected to be rewarded in terms of profit in return for their work. Both sides did what a number of different interest groups expected of them during the last decade before World War I.

Circumstances in DOA, primarily caused by the colonial system as such, made it impossible between 1890 and 1914 to solve the "labor problem" because irreconcilable differences existed between the parties concerned. There were also the ideological barriers imbedded in the political structure of DOA. At first labor problems were applicable only to agriculture. After 1900 they also affected employment in commerce, public works, and industry derived from agriculture. The question of labor was never solved but merely shifted to different levels. And in this process, government and industry proved to be more flexible than plantations and small farms. At no time did the settlers consider their supply of farm hands capable of supporting a healthy plantation system. Government and private non-agricultural employers changed their evaluation of the human potential of the African peasant during the last decade before World War I, even though they did not abandon their firm conviction that the economy of the dependent country was subsidiary to the economy of the colonial power. During the Rechenberg-Dernburg administration it was the peasant-laborer who derived temporary profit from the deadlocked struggle between the two sides. And the object of this struggle, the African peasant, improved his status although the improvements were motivated by predominantly egoistic considerations.[33] But at least, he was now protected from those settlers who advocated their own brand of "education for labor." "If we do not educate the blacks for labor," wrote DOAZ in 1908, "we shall educate them for disobedience." [34] Or, as von Geldern, chairman of the economic association of Rufiji wrote in an editorial in DOAZ in 1912, "should it really be called an injustice to compel the Negro . . . to cultivate larger tracts of land to make available for mankind the wealth hidden in the soil with all its promises of fertility?" [35] It would at least counteract the "negrophile excesses" of von Rechenberg whom the settlers held responsible for having taught the African not to work if he did not have to do so.[36] After Germany's departure from East Africa, German writers claimed that the loyal service of askaris and peasants during World War I was proof of Germany's good record as a colonial power. If so, it was true only where and when the Africans had been treated in a humane way.

German colonial social policy before 1914 did not stress the physical well-being of the millions of Africans it controlled as a separate factor in its program for labor. Health problems, however, turned up in policy considerations, whether wanted or not. They played a minor role under Wissmann and Schele. They became serious issues under von Götzen. Under Governors von Rechenberg and Schnee, the state stepped in and assumed responsibility for labor and health. Statistically, the outlook seemed unpromising. How could thirty-seven government doctors take care of ten million Africans? [37] Dr. Arning, retired staff medical officer, admitted in 1912 that the Reichstag might approve more funds for the medical service if pressed hard enough but the allocation of priorities was a matter of the Imperial Colonial Office "whose first and foremost duty it was to provide for the improvement of health." [38] Unfortunately medical care was only one among several obligations which competed for the limited budget of the Imperial Colonial Office. Apart from epidemics which required constant watchfulness, the personal health needs of the African could not be given the attention they received after World War I.

VI. MEDICINE, SCIENCE, AND SOCIETY TOWARD THE END OF GERMAN RULE IN EAST AFRICA

The impact of the colonial medical services on the welfare of labor in East Africa was not as significant as might be expected. Among other reasons, there was the fact that colonial policy lacked continuity and changed when it adjusted to different governors as well as different economic conditions. With the changes came different views of the character of "the African" and his potential for development. The planning for

---

[32] *Ibid.*, G12/208 Bl 190.
[33] Tetzlaff, *Koloniale Entwickelung*, p. 128.
[34] Dietrich Redeker, *Die Geschichte der Tagespresse Deutsch-Ostrafrikas*, p. 57.
[35] *Ibid.*, p. 61.
[36] *Ibid.*, p. 57. The labor law of March 23, 1910, had established minimum standards for working hours, living quarters, and nutrition.
[37] D Z St, R Kol A 1026, Bl 90.
[38] *Ibid.*, Bl 267.

the use of African manpower did only partially depend on rational considerations. Fluctuations in policy led to strange inconsistencies between observations derived from actual conditions in the country and actions taken upon recommendations by officials at home. Even the bureaucrats had to see that sick workers interfered with the progress of production. It was no secret that the volume of sisal production or the construction goals of railway mileage depended on the physical condition of the worker as much as on the equipment used for bridges and embankments. Wherever government assumed regulatory control over production, its attention was inevitably drawn to tribal society and the life style of the native worker.

Much closer to the people, by the very nature of their work, were the medical officials in the colonial service. Though not necessarily more interested in social and humanitarian issues or motivated by humanitarian considerations, they often became deeply involved in the exploration of the African background and the values that directed their lives. The same can be said of the scientists who changed their approach to their work. Called in by the government to help the planters produce better crops in spite of an adverse climate and damaging pests, they became increasingly more concerned with the task of exploring the nature of the environment as pure scientists. They did not abandon the original purpose of their work but as time went on it was overshadowed by pure research.

This trend was supported by the administrations of Governors Götzen, Rechenberg and Schnee who paid more attention to the pattern of life in African villages and the role of akidas as mediators between German officials and village communities. Special laboratories were approved to study plant seeds, soil and crop pests as well as animal and human diseases. Even the study of the physiology of nutrition and the hygiene of food habits was included. The Ministry of Health was prevailed upon and agreed to request additional funds of 15,409 marks in 1912 to hire two research specialists "to deal with the ever growing need to gain more knowledge of human metabolism and the transformation of caloric energy in natives and Europeans in tropical countries" in order to evaluate better the physiology of the African capacity for work.[1] Again, as many times before, this statement stressed economic utility as a measure-stick for the justification of scientific research but it also paved the way for pure research as such.

The changing climate of opinion is illustrated in an article published in *Koloniale Rundschau* in 1909. The writer rejected the old cherished gospel of the survival of the fittest as a justification for the support of the white community in DOA. Contrary to earlier theories which had attributed the absence of growth in Africa to the racial backwardness of the Negro who lacked the drive to create a civilization, this writer gave credit to the qualities of the African indigenous community. He called the black race the fittest to survive and to succeed in creating a viable economy in the tropics whereas he found the European "unfit" under the circumstances. Therefore he rejected the notion that in the highland districts the native race would have to make room for the white man as hypothetical and outright dangerous. The indigenous population, he wrote, was of extreme value to the colony and its agricultural production was indispensable to progress.[2] Such a startling turn-about, always of course within the framework of colonial paternalism, reflected years of experimentation based on the older theories. They were rejected when they could no longer be supported by the facts.

During the last decade before World War I the medical services in DOA continued conscientiously to take care of epidemics.[3] In their annual reports they listed action taken on intestinal and venereal diseases, leprosy, smallpox, tuberculosis, and sporadic outbreaks of cholera. Preventive medicine was given priority. But what was really done and what was merely declared as desirable? The statistics and even the description of cases do not give a clear picture. They list, for instance, the numbers of Africans who needed medical help in the stations of Bismarckburg, Neu Langenburg, Wilhelmstal. The report tells us of 13,241 sick people taken care of in 1903–1904 which may be typical or atypical since we do not know how many residents there were in the area.[4] They also listed the personnel employed by the services. Frequently they were satisfied with vague statements that in general the health of the population was good. Sometimes they discussed tribal characteristics in their reaction to medical treatment describing, for instance, the "free pastoral Wagaya" as more difficult to deal with and not responding to attempts at isolating them in sleeping sickness camps whereas other tribes used to dependence on authority could be more easily handled in medical emergencies. One does not know what conclusions they drew from their findings and what action was taken as a result.

If one were to rely exclusively on the official reports, the picture of health and disease in DOA would be very incomplete. The correspondence, resolutions, and complaints by public and private bodies reveal another side of the quality of the health services delivered by the colonial administration. There is the example of the Hamburg branch of German Colonial Society (DKG) whose resolution to the Executive Committee in May, 1912, openly expressed criticism of the colonial medical services and the administration. They compared the German medical services with those in neighboring territories and found progress in health in German colonies lagging. They noted a decline of

---

[1] TNA, G3/18, 110–115, 1912.

[2] "Die Entwickelung Deutsch-Ostafrikas im Jahre 1907/08," *Koloniale Rundschau* (1909), p. 198.

[3] See above chaps. 3 and 4.

[4] Z St A, R Kol A 1024, Bl 267/268 24 May, 1912.

the native population and recommended an increase in doctors, better community health care facilities like Tanga, Dar es Salaam, and Mombasa, a general upgrading of public health care, and more concern with such debilitating diseases as tuberculosis and venereal disease.

Former staff surgeon Dr. Arning and a member of the German Parliament in 1912 took a stand to the Hamburg resolution in a lengthy memorandum. He found it unsuitable for presentation to the Colonial Office because the latter was aware of its obligations to the colony and did not need the recital of obvious facts. "It was," he wrote, "the noblest task of colonial policy to stem the decline of the colored population; all sanitary work aimed in this direction and has had some success. Hasty efforts were not desirable whereas systematic action was the proper thing to do. And for this reason better training of doctors in public health institutes would have to be done in the future." After these generalities Dr. Arning answered specific points made by the Hamburg group. Community medical care was unsatisfactory only where self-government of the communes had been introduced. When the changeover came, the state withdrew its projects to leave it to the communities to do their own planning. Arning admitted that financial aid for medical services and public health should be subsidized by the government. Arning did not find fault with the government's program against tuberculosis which, he said, spread because of Indian immigration. He rejected a statement that the Colonial Office did not spend enough money for public health in the colonies. "After all," he wrote, "this work must be somehow in harmony with the progress of the overall development and with the financial capability of the entire budget."[5]

Arning's arguments against the memorandum were debatable. The petition was not drawn up as a blueprint for action on health care. Its purpose was merely to draw attention to the weakness of the system in order to bring about improvement. In view of Dr. Arning's past reputation in the colonial medical service and because of his political prestige at the time of the debate in the Colonial Society, he was the ideal person to stimulate reconsideration of medical and colonial policy and the broadening of its goals. Did he fear to antagonize Berlin and Dar es Salaam?

In October, 1913, a milder resolution was presented to the Executive Committee of DKG. It recommended the formation of a colonial medical advisory council similar to the British Colonial Medical Advisory Council in England. It asked for better health education of officials and for a government doctor in every district. It aimed at improvements not very different from those advocated by the Hamburg resolution. The advisory council would presumably have greater authority to give priority to public health and medical needs in spite of fiscal conservatism by the Colonial Office. The suggestion to place a doctor in every district would vastly enhance the quality of life of the African. This time the resolution which came from the Berlin branch of DKG was accepted for presentation to the Colonial Office. Since World War I broke out only one year later, it is impossible to know whether the medical services in DOA were ready to develop a new and broader program of preventive medicine tied to social services.[6] Spotty though these manifestations of criticism are, they show that by 1914 conservatives and professionals felt the need to push the Colonial Office toward an expansion of services which would reach the people in their villages.

If it were true that the government could not afford a larger budget for medical matters, why did it not make use of the medical missions to help in certain areas? One of the main reasons was that the relationship between government and missions was not a close one. The colonial government did not wish to finance mission medical work because it wanted to maintain a separation between private and public medical services. An attitude of watchful suspicion prevailed which was illustrated by a German "long-time resident in DOA, (a man) clearly striving to judge conditions objectively," when he analyzed the relationship between missions and government as follows: Government, he wrote in a Frankfurt newspaper in 1913, operates extensively from above, while missions operate intensively from below, from the bottom up. Government becomes involved in colonial affairs after military conquest. It remains the "superior master" (Grosser Herr) and rules with the aid of district officials. The missionary familiar with the customs and the language of those among whom he lives has much to contribute to government. But they seem to work at cross purposes. If the missionaries would stay out of politics, they would get along fine with the government. But the writer had reservations on whether the Church was the immediate and most pressing need of the colony. What the colonies needed most was education, not the Church. In the interest of harmonious cooperation which he found lacking, the author wished to assign distinct roles to each of the two partners.[7]

In government reports on medicine in DOA one barely reads about mission medical work during the earlier period. Governor Götzen gave the Foreign Office a list of missions active in the colony in 1904 and mentioned only two missions as having one doctor each on their staff.[8] Perhaps because of the small number of mission doctors or because of the centralization of power in the colony at the time, did the colonial administration not include medical missionaries as instrumental in its own scheme of operations. This attitude seems to emerge more clearly under Germany's first colonial secretary, Bernhard Dernburg. Although

---

[5] *Ibid.*, Bl 259, 260, 268.

[6] *Ibid.*, Bl 149/150.
[7] TNA, G9/4, Das Freie Wort, Frankfurt/Main, 1913, 89, 93.
[8] TNA, G9/2, Folder "Missions, General, 1904–1906," p. 7.

he would not subsidize medical missions or promote their growth in DOA, he tried to maintain friendly relations without becoming obligated to them. This led to conflicting statements on different occasions. When Privy Counsellor Berner, an upper administrative court judge and official rapporteur for the missions with the German Colonial Office, corresponded with Dernburg in 1907 on mission complaints in Moshi, Dernburg made a thorough examination of the charges. Lieutenant Abel, the military chief of the station in Moshi, gave examples which showed that seven Lutheran Evangelical missions and three Catholic missions of the Catholic Black Fathers saturated the area with their presence. Catholics and Protestants struggled among themselves and with the government. The Africans in the district tolerated them only because they feared unfavorable action by the military. The missions coerced the Africans into accepting their orders and their way of living. They acted like a quasi government (Nebenregierung) disregarding government regulations. They were only concerned with their immediate objective to get the people into their Church and did not care for the long-range plans of the government. In this case Dernburg agreed with the report of his official in the field and dismissed any accusations made by the missions that they were under the tyranny of a military coercive system. He requested that the Lutheran mission publicly withdraw its accusations in the official organ of the Lutheran mission.[9] The incident in itself was not important. Friction between missions and government occurred throughout the period in German and English colonies. In spite of his more liberal views and his preference of civilian officials in colonial service, Dernburg upheld and defended in this case the military administrators of Moshi and exonerated them. He found that they had acted entirely within their rights and in the interest of the African population.

The problem became more complex in the case of medical mission services. Here the administrators were torn between two conflicting choices. They wanted to increase the number of non-governmental and non-military doctors whose salary would not have to be paid by the imperial treasury, but they also wanted to maintain absolute control over medical training and medical performance. One notices this controversial stand in the actions and declarations by officials and professionals, especially during the last ten years of German rule in DOA.

After his return from East Africa in 1907 Dernburg declared, "a system of medical care for the black man does not at present exist, as far as government is concerned. I believe that it is here where missions will find a very rewarding field in which to operate. ... The extremely high mortality rate in East Africa makes the absence of proper provisions for medical care for the native a real emergency." He requested to be kept informed of the progress of medical training for missionaries in Tübingen giving a clear mandate for action.[10] But action had to wait while professionals and bureaucrats continued their discussions. Dr. Steudel, a former senior staff surgeon with the *Schutztruppe* and later in the German Colonial Office, acknowledged in 1909 that there were too few doctors in the colonies for the huge territory that had to be covered and that was so densely populated.[11] Still another report illustrates the urgency of the problem of doctors. The chairman of the medical missionary association in Leipzig gave a grim description to the executive committee of the German Colonial Society in 1910. Dr. Ittameier, a recently appointed doctor of the Evangelical Lutheran mission in Kilimanjaro, Pare, and Meru, faced an almost unsurmountable workload from the very beginning of his medical work. Hundreds of Africans who had been without a doctor for several years needed his help.

Marching for days at a time through the savanna and through mountainous territory taxed the power and the resistance of the doctor. According to his statistical account for the quarter from August to October, 1909, 385 cases had been treated [under these difficult circumstances], a clear proof that the station was in dire need of a doctor in the area.[12]

There was a rare unanimity among all those concerned with medical matters that relief for the medical personnel in DOA was urgent. Nevertheless, the missions had great trouble in obtaining government subsidies when they began to plan for an enlarged medical service. Missions had been slow in increasing their medical staff in East Africa after 1901 when the colony began to function in a more orderly way. There is no doubt that they were aware of the exceedingly important role which medical missions were able to fulfill if properly staffed. After all, David Livingstone's first trip to South Africa in 1841 was the direct result of the recognition of the medical factor in missionary work. But for decades the missions did not separate their religious work from their medical operations, nor did they have large enough funds to put a doctor into every mission. After 1905 they formed medical missionary associations to cope with the increasing need for medical work. This came at a time of commercial expansion and the improvement of internal communications. Before the end of the century, there had been only one society for medical missions, the Stuttgart medical missionary association founded in 1899. A much more comprehensive development started with the establishment in Tübingen in 1906 of an institute of medical missions for all German and Swiss evangelical mission societies. Its purpose was to dispatch doctors

---

[9] TNA, G9/32 Dernburg to Berner, 12 March, 1907, p. 30.

[10] Z St A, R Kol A 1026, Bl 11, Dernburg to Berner, November 23, 1907.

[11] *Archiv für Schiffs-und Tropenhygiene* (1909), Dr. Steudel, "Der ärztliche Dienst in den deutschen Schutzgebieten," p. 29.

[12] Z St A, R Kol A, 1026, Bl 90.

to the colonies and to train them for this purpose.[13] It was supplemented by medical mission associations in the Rhineland in 1906 and five more associations in Berlin, Braunschweig, Halle, Leipzig, and Munich in 1908.[14] Though doctors had been connected with missions for a long time and had been actively recruited by them, neither the training seminars for missionaries at home nor the stations in the field had made a concerted effort to plan for the continued flow of medical personnel wherever it was needed.[15] The medical service at missions was in the majority of cases limited to paraprofessional work by wives of missionaries, nurses, and the missionaries themselves who treated emergencies and concerned themselves with infant care, lighter surgical cases, and first aid. They made inroads in gaining the confidence of the Africans living in their midst but they could not even contemplate the major problem of preventive and curative medicine.

This was the situation when in 1908 another major step was contemplated by both the missions and the government. The institute for medical missions in Tübingen asked the German Colonial Society for financial help in order to go ahead with a much needed building for the education of mission doctors. The request was denied after lengthy discussions. A similar resolution reintroduced in 1909 and 1910 reveals the fears and suspicions on both sides. The Society wanted a clear definition of the term "mission doctor." If he was a "real" physician, it was up to the government to train him and the Society need not be concerned with the problem. Some debaters even questioned the need for the mission's medical institute building. Consul Vohsen, prominent member of the Board, thought money should be spent on more important things and wanted the mission's request referred to the Colonial Office. One of the Society's directors was dissatisfied with the vagueness of the request as presented. He wanted to know where the mission doctors would operate and under what regulations.[16] A year later in May, 1909, the situation had changed slightly. The building for the training of mission doctors had been completed and pastor Thiessen, the mission spokesman, asked for 30,000 marks to operate it. Consul Vohsen was as categorical as he was a year before and declared that a subsidy of 30,000 marks was out of the question. This time the objections by the Society were clearly defined. One, missionary doctors must not compete with civilian doctors. Two, missionary doctors must not propagandize the work of their mission. Three, mission doctors must be subject to the rules and regulations of the protectorate.[17] The board of the association for medical missions was unperturbed and approached the Society again in August, 1910, with a request for help which was supported by the presentation of substantial evidence. This time acceptance of the mission's request for a subsidy was recommended.[18] Dependence by mission fund-raisers on the good will of the powerful commercial and plantation interests of DKG should not lead to the conclusion that mission doctors themselves occupied a lesser role in the colony. Drs. Ittameier and Feldmann, both active as missionary doctors in DOA before 1914, were accepted as professionally competent. Both wrote scholarly demographic studies on the indigenous population in DOA. The publication of their studies was sponsored by the German Colonial Institute of Hamburg.[19] Nevertheless, the policy of separate but equal remained in force to the end.

This impression is supported by several papers presented at meetings of the Hamburg and German society for tropical medicine in 1908 and 1909. Dr. König, for instance, a retired naval staff surgeon general, accepted the associations for medical missions as desirable and asked only for a clear separation of duties. He expected that the medical associations should have absolute control over the health and medical activities of the mission doctors, leaving to the missions only responsibility for their general objectives.[20] Others went much farther. They wanted a clean-cut separation between the profession of the doctor and the work of the missionary. Professor Schilling, director of tropical diseases and tropical hygiene at the Institute for Infectious Diseases in Berlin, said,

we do not want to, and we cannot, prevent a colleague from practicing his Christian convictions when he advises those patients who ask for his advice on the Christian religion. But I cannot approve of an association which selects and trains doctors and sends them out with the obligation ... to promote the goals of the missions directly and indirectly. ... I cannot recommend to a younger colleague to become dependent on an association whose members are largely laymen, an association, moreover, which gives the missions a decisive voice.[21]

He preferred instead an association advised by doctors who would also be responsible for the medical training of their mission students. Missionary financial support of these associations would entitle them to get the doctors they needed. Dr. Schilling's view was supported by another member, Dr. Kirchner from Berlin, who stressed the fact that he was brought up in a preacher's home and had always been fond of missions. But then he asked the rhetorical question "what does the mission have to do with the doctor?" and implied a negative

---

[13] *Deutsches Kolonialblatt* 20, 1909, "Der ärztliche Dienst in den deutschen Schutzgebieten," p. 970.
[14] Z St A, R Kol A, Bl 1026, Bl 2.
[15] *Deutsches Kolonialblatt*, "Arztliche Mission," **19** (1908): p. 72.
[16] Z St A, R Kol A, 1026, Bl 42–46.
[17] *Ibid.*, Bl 112–114.
[18] *Ibid.*, Bl 126.
[19] Hamburgische Universität, *Wissenschaftliche Beiträge zur Frage der Erhaltung und Vermehrung der Eingeborenen-Bevölkerung*, Dr. med Carl Ittameier, pp. 1–82; Dr. med Hermann Feldmann, pp. 83–144.
[20] *Archiv*, 1908, Harry Koenig, Arztliche Mission und Tropenhygiene, p. 113.
[21] *Ibid.*, Claus Schilling, Über den ärztlichen Dienst in den deutschen Schutzgebieten, p. 38.

answer. He advised the Society for Tropical Medicine not to support the associations for medical missionaries because it was impossible for mission doctors to be fully independent in any dispute between doctor and mission since decisions were made by the superintendent of the mission.[22]

The passion of the debates was remarkable. Was dependence on a Christian mission worse than dependence on the state or the military? It appears that at this time the majority of the medical profession favored state support and state control for medical education for doctors in the colonies even though they complained about the inadequacy of medical budgets. This, they hoped, could be remedied by influencing the colonial government and the public and by making them understand the value of medicine in the colonies. Dr. Schilling, moreover, disagreed with the assumption that the missionary had a closer relationship with the African than the doctor. He saw the doctor as mediator between black and white and regretted that the doctor's potentially valuable services in this respect were not properly utilized by the government. But regardless of the dispute on the relative advantages of the mission doctor over the government doctor or vice versa, the medical profession was closer to the population in its everyday affairs than other government officials. The doctors reported on diseases, inherited traits and customs affecting disease, and, in spite of racial bias and racial prejudice, they could not help but draw conclusions from their findings. Their thinking might be influenced by preconceived notions on the nature of the African as expressed in the earlier years of German rule. But by the end of the period one notices that even the more inflexible minds admitted their ignorance of African customs and traditions and their wish to understand them better.

It is these reactions to the phenomena experienced locally and to observations over a longer period of time that yielded results. Dr. Ittameier prefaced his essay on the causes of infant mortality and population decline in DOA with some general observations on the problem of gaining access to the African. "Why was it so difficult," he asked, "to get truthful statements about family life among the natives?" His answer was that lying had become their second nature. He modified this shocking statement by a rationalized explanation. The Negro, he said, lies because he fears that truthful answers might bring some unknown damaging repercussions or that his kinsmen might hold cooperation with the European against him, or that the Europeans might use the information in a way that would endanger him and his family. There was, according to him, a lack of confidence which stemmed in part from the long and slow process of pacification in the colony. Ittameier concluded that "today [i.e., 1920] we are still absolutely unable to obtain useful information from some tribes. . . . Only a smaller number of tribes remains from whom we have obtained more accurate information." [23]

But it was possible to establish contact with the African and even a working relationship. This was true in the case of sleeping sickness and leprosy which required segregation of the sick from the remainder of the population. Doctors were able to gain the confidence of the people to treat them against infectious and spreading disease, such as venereal diseases, tuberculosis, and smallpox. They made less headway in the battle against infant mortality, aborted births, and worm diseases because their treatment required a change of their ways of living. Medical care, whether undertaken for selfish or lofty reasons, expedited the search for an understanding of the African way of life although it did not succeed in changing it when it was necessary to do so for medical reasons. But as was seen before,[24] it is unfair to judge the German medical achievements in DOA as they were in 1917. The major success in colonial medicine occurred after World War I.

In his analysis of the impact of western culture on African life, Ittameier placed major emphasis on the consequences of land alienation, on labor recruitment of Africans away from their home and families, and on the difference of customs, beliefs, and superstitions which made it difficult for western man to grasp the mind of the African. For instance, he found that among the Chagga of Kilimanjaro five-sixths of all infants died during the first four years of their lives while only one-sixth survived into later years. This figure did not include abortions which he estimated at somewhere between 10 and 16 per cent.[25] Why did government and missions not do more to reduce infant mortality? Ittameier gave several reasons. Western contacts created better communications, built railways, brought better methods of production, all of which led to greater mobility and thereby facilitated the spread of disease without presenting the African with a sufficient number of doctors to take care of the increased health hazards. More than one doctor should have been stationed at government and mission centers. But those who planned for commercial and industrial expansion did not at first rank public health and medicine among the top priorities. The changes which DOA experienced in the course of development made the women the most vulnerable targets. Ittameier found fault with the expansion of European settlements at the expense of the African. He also deplored the absence of educational campaigns against superstition and animistic beliefs which should have accompanied the introduction of public health.[26]

---

[22] *Ibid.*, G. Olpp, Das deutsche Institut für ärztliche Mission, Discussion, p. 67.

[23] *Hamburgische Universität, Wissenschaftliche Abhandlungen*, Ittameier, p. 4.
[24] See above chap. 2.
[25] Ittameier, *op. cit.*, p. 38.
[26] *Ibid.*, pp. 59–64.

In his treatment of civilization and its impact on African life, Feldmann came to similar conclusions. He found the African peasants in a disadvantaged position because of the dangers which affected their health and their continued growth. Customs which led to a high rate of abortions and ignorance which caused an abnormally high number of infant deaths affected their future. "This [preexisting] unfavorable situation," he wrote, "is aggravated by the unavoidable penetration into African life of a European culture which brings with it much that is dangerous, in addition to other aspects in European civilization which are good, and threatens the African more in his fight for survival than was the case before."[27] Feldmann placed the responsibility for the improvement of the health of the African and his survival in the future on the colonial government, the missionaries, and the settlers. Both Feldmann and Ittameier believed that it was possible to create better living conditions for the African within the framework of the colonial system.

One theme was central in the deliberations on the creation of a more suitable environment for the people in DOA. This was the use of science as a weapon and an aid in the battle against disease among plants and men. Scientists had been responsible for research on tropical disease. Scientists had assisted planters in analyzing crop failures; they had fought against animal disease. In 1900 the Colonial Economic Committee (KWK) reaffirmed its conviction that the German colonies were bound to become in time a valuable factor within the German economic system. In the pursuit of this goal, the Committee adopted a program (1) to promote the production of tropical food products and technologically valuable raw materials needed for the home market up to an estimated total of one billion marks, (2) to study the production and preparation of crops in foreign economic areas, and (3) to educate the German people on the status and needs of their colonial economy.[28] To achieve these goals the Committee scrutinized the causes of failures in agricultural production and commercial enterprises in the colony and recommended the creation of an agricultural research station which would apply science and research to the very practical end of making colonial enterprises more profitable. It also approached the Foreign Office and the colonial administration with a request to support their plan.

The German Africanist Detlev Bald has emphasized that the initiative for what was to become the biological and agricultural institute at Amani was taken by KWK, and not by the German government. The pragmatic character of research was, therefore, the primary motive in conducting scientific research at Amani.[29]

This may be correct to a certain extent but the German government and the colonial administration had supported research for a long time in their battle against tropical disease. Laboratories had been set up for Robert Koch's experimentation with rats and mosquitoes in the 1890's to curb cholera and malaria. But a new role for research in colonial DOA was indicated when Governor Götzen described the scope and function of the new biological and agricultural institute by proclamation in 1902. The institute was set up on African soil as a permanent facility. It was given a separate professional staff trained in botany, chemistry, geology, and mineralogy.[30] Yet it was only a beginning. It still had to go a long way before reaching the status of a full-fledged research organization. Without the active support of KWK, however, it might never have got off the ground at that particular period of DOA's development. The planters themselves, the beneficiaries of the institute, had too narrow an orientation toward immediate tangible results to serve as proper midwives for Amani's birth.

After their 1900 meeting KWK sent Dr. Otto Warburg, one of its co-founders in 1896 and a professor of botany at the University of Berlin, on an exploratory trip to several of the established research institutes maintained by the English, Dutch, French, and Belgian tropical colonies. In his report to the German Colonial Congress in 1902 Warburg strongly supported the application of theoretical research to the practical pursuit of colonial problems. His presentation paid tribute to Germany's past scientific achievements which as a newcomer was the last of the colonial powers to set up a scientific institute in the tropical colonies. "No other nation in the world," he said, "had as thoroughly conquered its colonies with the aid of science, as the Germans had done and this included not only natural science, zoology, botany, geography, ethnology, and the related sciences of anthropology, meteorology, climatology, etc. but also the medical sciences and . . . linguistics, jurisprudence, and folklore."[31] Why did Warburg plead for a new central institute of research supported by the state if, as he said, the sciences had not only accompanied colonial activity but even preceded it? His answer was that there were no scientific organizations for the theoretical study of problems of the colonial economy and he urged that economic development be placed on a scientific basis. It was Warburg, the representative of German industrialists, who pleaded for the marriage of science and industry. But he also warned that the colony had reached the stage at which the Colonial Economic Committee alone could no longer cope with the continuous need for new inventions like better devices for harvesting, better meth-

---

[27] Feldmann, *op. cit.*, p. 143.

[28] *Das Deutsche Kolonialblatt* (1900), Kolonialwirtschaftliches Komitee, p. 560.

[29] Detlev Bald, Das Forschungsinstitut AMANI (München, 1972), pp. 27-29.

[30] *Deutsches Kolonialblatt* (1902), Bekanntmachung betreffend die Verwaltung des Biologisch-Landwirtschaftlichen Instituts zu Amani, pp. 433, 434.

[31] *Verhandlungen des Deutschen Kolonialkongresses* (1902), Dr. Otto Warburg, pp. 193, 195.

ods for the processing of rubber, a more intensive system of tsetse and insect control, the improvement of oil palm cultures and many other colonial commodities. To insure the continuity of the diverse programs undertaken by KWK, he suggested the creation of an independent institute to pursue practical problems, based on scientific investigations. Once in existence, the institute should be operated by the state. And this is what happened in 1902. After several years, however, it changed its character more than Warburg may have anticipated although at first it accepted the principles suggested by KWK. Paragraph two of the guidelines for Amani issued by Governor Götzen in 1902 directed the institute to serve the practical needs of DOA in every possible way. No expenses were to be incurred for scientific tasks not directly connected with the improvement and preservation of the agricultural and industrial economy of the colony.[32] This included not only the European but especially the African population. The institute's assignments included investigations of conditions of growth in tropical plants, the control of agents causing animal and plant disease, analyses of the soil, and related matters. A professional staff was in charge of laboratories for botany, zoology, mineralogy, and geology. The institute's first annual report in 1903 stated again that research was limited to the useful role which plants played in the development of the colony.[33] Accordingly, Amani promoted research on rubber, cotton, coffee, and sisal. Only cotton and sistal justified the economic investment through research because they did not decline in value on the world market as did rubber and coffee in 1914.[34]

An important aspect of Amani, the education of planters and settlers in better methods of cultivation, proved to be more difficult than expected. Many of the planters were not professionals, nor were they prepared for their work in the colony. They could not make use of professional advice which Amani had to offer and were irritated by unsolicited interference. And even those who were trained as agronomists had never been in touch with scientific institutes at home.[35] One vital prerequisite, therefore, for the success of applied research, the cooperation between the staff of Amani and the men in the field, remained practically unfulfilled. Scientists like Zimmermann, Vossler, Stuhlmann, and Lommel produced results of greatest value. They were praised at the Colonial Congress in 1910 as having essentially contributed to the agricultural advancement of DOA. It was pointed out that their work had proven how infinitely more financially rewarding their research had been to the entire colony than the entire cost of the operations at Amani.[36] This was said by Professor Volkens, the custodian of the central botanical office for the colonies in Berlin, and shows that eight years after the foundation of Amani even scientists found it necessary to stress again and again the argument of the ultimate economic profit to be derived from pure research. The general public and the leaders in agriculture and industry seemed to have remained skeptical.

Secretary of State for the Colonies, Dr. Wilhelm Solf, confirmed this view in 1912 on his tour of DOA. He was impressed by Amani and saw it finally reaching the level of Buitenzorg, the Dutch agricultural research institute on Java which had served as a model for Amani in 1902. He proposed to raise Amani's budget of 60,000 marks and castigated the planters "who, here too, demonstrated their hostility to the scholars" and did not want to admit the importance of scientific investigations without which the practical work of the plantations could not be carried out.[37]

But what about medical research? Amani was expressly limited to the natural sciences, exclusive of medicine. There is essential evidence to assume that if the Germans had remained in DOA beyond 1917, they most likely would have established an institute for tropical medicine in one of their African colonies, preferably in Dar es Salaam. This institute, contrary to the pragmatism which dominated Amani, would have been dedicated from the outset exclusively to scientific and medical research on tropical medicine and tropical hygiene. The discussion on such an institute was held at the meeting of the Society for Tropical Medicine in Berlin in 1909. Many different views were presented, and in spite of differences of opinion, there was no real disagreement. What makes this discussion so interesting and almost contemporary, certainly not dated, is the clear presentation of the essentials of scientific research which must be free from bureaucratic control and permit the formulation of themes for investigation solely on the merit of the problem regardless of practical considerations.

The major topics discussed in connection with a future tropical institute for medical research centered on its location, its size, its source of control, and the total range of its research but not on the need of an institute as such. It was generally postulated and accepted that tropical diseases must be studied in the tropical country where they occurred. The excellent facilities in Berlin, Hamburg, Tübingen, and elsewhere where tropical diseases were studied and where much research had been done for decades did not invalidate the need for a colonial tropical research institute in

---

[32] *Deutsches Kolonialblatt* (1902), Bekanntmachung, p. 433.
[33] *Ibid.*, 1903, p. 677.
[34] See economic statistics.
[35] *Denkschrift über die Entwickelung der deutschen Schutzgebiete* (Berlin 1905/06). Cited by Bald, Das Forschungsinstitut Amani, p. 80.

[36] D. G. Volkens, Die Entwickelung des auf wissenschaftlicher Grundlage ruhenden landwirtschaftlichen Versuchswesens in den Kolonien, *Verhandlungen des Deutschen Kolonialkongresses* (1910), p. 67.
[37] Solf Papers (Nachlass Solf), /36. Observations on trip through East Africa, 25 August, 1912, p. 76.

medicine. Dr. Schilling, himself the director of the department of tropical diseases in Berlin, made this point very clear before going into further detail of tropical medical research. In a memorandum to the colonial secretary in 1908 and at a meeting of the Society for Tropical Medicine in 1909, he described the basic structure of a colonial institute devoted to research in tropical medicine. His broad and generous outline far surpassed the much narrower points made by his discussants. The institute as he envisaged it must be open to research specialists in many fields like bacteriology, parasitology, physiology, hygiene, and veterinary medicine. It must have the facilities needed for work, including laboratories and supporting manpower. It must be open to universities, academies, scientific institutes, the *Schutztruppe,* and younger academicians. And since it was planned on such a broad scale, it must be financed by the government.[38] The discussion on his plan did not indicate disagreement with the core of his proposals. It is, however, indicative that the German official publication *Deutsches Kolonialblatt* of 1909 in reviewing Schilling's presentation admitted that there was agreement on the creation of an institute but emphasized general disagreement regarding the magnitude of Schilling's plan. Officials judged the feasibility of his presentation from a purely budgetary point of view.[39]

Apart from minor objections, one issue encountered more opposition. Schilling stressed in uncompromising terms the exclusively scientific functions of the institute and its complete operational independence from the colonial administration. Several doctors attacked him as too impractical and utopian. Dr. Plehn, chief surgeon of a major hospital in Berlin, was equally emphatic in wishing to place the research institute within the structure of colonial government and administration. How could it function, he asked, if it was not supported by the administrators on the spot? Academic and scientific objectives could not be achieved, he argued, if the institute were placed outside the hierarchy of the colonial medical department.

Even though there was a great sense of urgency in the discussion, a resolution to the Colonial Office in Berlin was not drafted at the meeting in 1909. The magnitude of the proposal was fully grasped by everyone but the consensus was that more soul-searching was needed. A humorous participant suggested that everyone return to the privacy of his chamber and meditate quietly. Dr. Bernard Nocht of the Hamburg Institute for Tropical Medicine suggested that no further report on the proposal be made for another five years. Thus the medical elite assembled at Berlin in 1909 went home with a good conscience, satisfied that it had contributed a good discussion to a worthy cause. The colonial medical administration of DOA remained without a tropical research institute in medicine in East Africa until the outbreak of World War I which does not imply that research in tropical medicine had been abandoned. On the contrary, it was taken very seriously as was shown before.[40]

By 1914 the medical profession was remarkably frank in its evaluation of its achievements. Its major criticism was directed at the lack of personnel which prevented the steady growth of a balanced program of curative and preventive medicine. It also admitted that it had not done enough for the bulk of the population. During the earlier years government officials and doctors had discussed this issue in terms of enlightened self-interest. During the Rechenberg-Schnee administrations concern for the indigenous population was defended in a more sophisticated way. It now reflected the argument of humanitarianism, the recognition that a tropical colony could not function without the native population adjusted to the climate, and the awareness that a composite industrial-agricultural economy must be based on the bulk of the population rather than an imported minority. If it was the task of the colonial economy in general to activate the individual Negro fully, it was the duty of the colonial public health service to activate the totality of the economic forces represented by the indigenous population, to maintain their vitality and their productivity.[41] This was the way in which government surgeon Külz justified his concern with the indigenous population in 1910. Dr. Peiper, a senior staff surgeon of the *Schutztruppe* in DOA combined a larger dose of ethics with the customary economic arguments in an article in 1911. He viewed with anxiety the appalling statistics of infant mortality in DOA and urged that something be done about it immediately. "It must be our most noble task," he wrote, "to preserve a large, healthy and diligent Negro population in our colonies. For the most precious asset of our possessions are not diamonds, minerals, plantations and large numbers of wild animals but 'man as such.' Not only has the colonial power the ethical and moral obligation to preserve man in Africa, but the practical interest of the state demands it just as well." [42]

Various formulations of similar humanitarian-utilitarian thoughts can be found in the discussions on public health, problems of population growth, the causes of the failure of medicine to penetrate to the social core of the African. But relatively little was said before 1920 about the most intriguing problem of native policy, namely its ability or inability to preserve tribal life while trying simultaneously to bring western civilization closer to the African. The problem was recognized but not yet given priority to be dealt with as a

---

[38] Claus Schilling, Uber den ärztlichen Dienst, *Archiv* (1909), p. 43.
[39] *Deutsches Kolonialblatt* (1909), p. 970.
[40] See above pp. 34, 35.
[41] Dr. Külz, *Wesen und Ziele der Eingeborenenhygiene in den deutschen Kolonien, Kolonialkongress* (1910), p. 346.
[42] Otto Peiper, "Die v. Pirquetsche Kutane Tuberkulinreaktion," *Archiv* (1911), p. 23.

separate issue. Colonial Secretary Bernhard Dernburg presented some ideas on native policy to the German Parliament in 1908. He had found that the more successful government was in developing the colony, the more it was compelled to face a new problem. Development increased demands on the native population to participate in the economy and thereby forced it to change its way of life, its working habits, its response to taxation, and imposed on it judicial procedures not contained in tribal law. Frictions were likely to develop which should make the colonizing power pause and consider the consequences. Would not the rising demands it made diminish the favorable position it had gained? And like Dr. Külz he admonished the members of Parliament that the most important asset in Africa was the indigenous African.[43]

Others addressed themselves to the more concrete problems of the same issues. In 1909 an official medical report on the plague in Dar es Salaam analyzed the topography of the city and the habits of its non-European inhabitants in a factual analysis without, however, giving a clue to remedial measures. The report stressed African indolence, especially among Islamic Negroes who did not show concern with matters that did not affect them personally in a direct way.[44] It was not impossible to deal with the plague diagnostically, but it presented enormous problems as a social issue. To eliminate the hiding places of rats which harbored the plague bacillus, the natives would have to be forced out of their houses and into a new pattern of living. Therefore, one was satisfied with campaigns against rats which Koch had begun in 1896. The number of rats killed by 1912 was listed as 170,000. Yet, no account was given of people who had changed from mud huts to healthier types of houses. Was the task considered too costly or self-defeating? Ernst Marshall, a former senior staff physician, wrote in 1924 that Germany's record in its treatment of natives was good. The colonial doctor had gained the confidence of the African with whom he often established a close relationship. He fulfilled his mission, according to Marshall, out of humanitarian reasons and lived up to the obligations of every civilized nation towards those who were still on a lower cultural level.[45]

Not the doctor, but the missionary, concerned himself more deeply with the nature of the African and his ability to accept values which would help western officials to make his protégé accept a new outlook on life. At the Colonial Congress in 1910 a German Protestant minister outlined the problem of "the soul of the Negro" and how it affected the chances of his development. Though he loaded his report with contemporary racial concepts, the minister came to the conclusion that the Negro's ability to learn and to change had been proven over the years. Dr. Külz, former government physician in the Cameroons, was much more critical in this respect and would admit only that western influence was capable of educating the Negro for work without changing his cultural level, although he emphasized that he had enjoyed close and cordial relationships with his Negro patients. The debate on the report of the Protestant minister showed that only a small minority was willing to grant that the African was capable of adjusting to western civilization. Whether the postwar era might have led to a new approach in the relationship between the colonial government and its African population remains a purely speculative issue. Generally speaking, the Africans in DOA profited from the attention of their medical protectors. But they had only reached the first stage toward emancipation from the arbitrariness of the hostile forces of tropical nature when World War I broke out and caused a considerable setback.

VII. WORLD WAR I AND ITS IMPACT ON PEOPLE, POLITICS, AND HEALTH

Historical evaluations of General von Lettow Vorbeck's military operations in DOA have produced tendentious, embittered, apologetic, appreciative, and recently a few well-balanced analyses. The period has been covered widely in monographs and in general histories. The war in itself is not the subject of this chapter. Participants in the war, settlers, military writers, and friends as well as foes of the German colonial regime in East Africa have praised the general's military abilities and his extreme sense of duty which bordered on fanaticism, qualities which enabled him to hold out with his small force against a larger British army in the surrounding colonies.[1] They have analyzed Lettow Vorbeck's contribution to the total war effort. They have been critical of the slow response by the British forces to counter the German offensive in the Kilimanjaro district and the extended harassment of British forces by Lettow's soldiers, even after General Smuts had taken over the command of the King's African Rifles. And finally much attention has been paid to Lettow's sustained guerilla warfare between 1917 and 1918 long after Smuts declared the war as ended as far as British assignments were concerned. The fact that Lettow Vorbeck did not surrender immediately when the armistice was announced on November 11, 1918, but held his position until the twenty-fifth of the month, was due as much to British fair play in DOA as to Lettow Vorbeck's dogged stubbornness to

---

[43] Dernburg, Fragen der Eingeborenenpolitik, *Deutsches Kolonialblatt* (1908), pp. 217, 218.
[44] *Archiv* (1910), p. 3.
[45] Ernst Morshall, Ärztlicher Dienst und ärztliche Forschung in den deutschen Kolonien, *Das Deutsche Kolonialbuch* (1926), p. 117.

[1] For books on Lettow Vorbeck and the war see: Lettow Vorbeck, *Meine Erinnerungen aus Ostafrika* (1921). Ludwig Boell, *Die Operationen in Ost Afrika*. Heinrich Loth, *Griff nach Ostafrika*, Ludwig Deppe, *Mit Lettow Vorbeck durch Afrika*, Maximilian Decher, *Afrikanisches und Allzu-Afrikanisches*, and others in the bibliography.

maintain what he considered the honor of the German army. But neither his bearing during the war nor British reaction to Lettow Vorbeck's military campaigns influenced the political future of Tanganyika. It was decided by many factors which shall be briefly discussed in this chapter.

Lettow Vorbeck arrived in Dar es Salaam in January, 1914, and had little time before war broke out to familiarize himself with the country. He could not explore the African social structure, its tribal characteristics and the diverse responses by Africans to the demands made on them by settlers and officials. He was, however, aware of potential frictions and mentioned in his book on the war that some fear of a native rising had been expressed in many quarters, especially among the Wahehe along the central railway and near Iringa, the site of the 1905 Maji Maji revolt. He also reported that the authorities had reservations about the large numbers of black laborers on European farms which represented an element of danger. But he hoped that African opinion was well expressed by an English Masai who had said, "It is all the same to us whether the English or the Germans are our masters." [2] In deciding on a strategy, however, he was solely influenced by his own observations. He drew conclusions from the wealth of cattle among the Masai and trusted that it would supply his army even if he were cut off from overseas supplies. He admired the lush and fertile agricultural districts he found in the north near his Kilimanjaro stronghold where many fields had been abandoned by the natives who had moved on to newer fields. He ventured to predict unlimited possibilities of development in East Africa.[3] The spirit displayed by the askari impressed him although he regretted that their German sergeants had trained them poorly. His observations were quite different from those of the administrators who, under Rechenberg and Schnee, had come to the conclusion that German East Africa was not a place for European settlers and for further immigration and that its future would have to depend on crops produced by the Africans themselves.

Not burdened, therefore, by apprehensions of revolts, labor shortages and insufficient numbers of carriers and porters, Lettow Vorbeck conceived his plan of continuously threatening the British in their own territory, forcing them to maintain their defensive ability in the African theater of war where they had not intended to wage active warfare. Governor Schnee who was familiar with the labor problems of the past and who knew the risk involved in separating the men from their village communities for longer periods of time disagreed with Lettow Vorbeck on his plan of an aggressive war on East African soil.

Ludwig Boell, personal adjutant to Lettow Vorbeck throughout the war, gave a vivid description of his superior's iron determination to carry out his master plan. It was based on a policy of sustained attack and unceasing harassment. He decided to shift his pattern of attack constantly and required an instant adjustment by his own officers to the rapidly changing character of his maneuvers which taxed the stamina of his European personnel to the extreme. Obsessed by his plan of relentless harassment of the enemy, he found himself increasingly isolated by his own staff.[4] His drive and his example transformed his Protective Force into an elite corps. Weaker elements were dropped or left voluntarily and morale became better the longer the war lasted.[5]

But even though Boell described Lettow Vorbeck's relationship with his African soldiers as good, he admitted that the men knew they were not fighting for their own cause. They felt their treatment was just in spite of the sacrifices they had to endure, he wrote. He described the attitude of Lettow Vorbeck's army during the war as "in one word: above all praise. We felt as safe in East Africa during the war as in Abraham's lap, so to speak. There was no one who doubted the attitude of the natives for even one minute." [6]

How does one account for this African loyalty during a colonial war which deprived many of the people of their livelihood and their accustomed way of life? Was it the military presence which prevented an uprising? Boell explained African loyalty to the army as stemming from the German prewar policy which he labeled as correct and strict. The use of the whip and twenty-five strokes on their behind, carried out with the meticulous precision so characteristic of Prussian sergeants, was interpreted by Boell as not inhumane if compared with the uncertainty of arbitrary punishment which was not clearly defined in advance. At least the African knew what he had to expect when he misbehaved and when he was punished in the known and accustomed way, he felt that he was treated justly. Implied in this view was the acceptance of the right of the state to act in an authoritarian way in *loco parentis* and this again was based on the colonial concept that the protecting power was obligated to act as a father toward his ward, the immature African native. The western concept of trial by jury and the prohibition of corporeal punishment was judged inappropriate under the circumstances.

Like other historians Boell acknowledged that the eight million Africans who endured the war in DOA were exposed to its horror and felt the brunt of tropical warfare. They suffered through famines and disease without using the war as an opportunity to revolt

---

[2] *Lettow Vorbeck*, p. 28.
[3] *Ibid.*, pp. 8–9.
[4] Ludwig Boell, *Die Operationen in Ost-Afrika*, p. 431.
[5] Maximilian Decher who spent the entire war in the ranks under Lettow Vorbeck gave a less favorable picture of African support. "Most of the tribes of our colonies, whether in the Lake Nyanza or Tanganyika area, near Tabora, in the highlands of Iringa, near Kilimanjaro or in the south near the coast ... were already in times of peace ill-disposed." *Afrikanisches und Allzu-Afrikanisches*, p. 283.
[6] Boell, Communication to the author, February 2, 1975.

against the colonial regime. There are no authentic reports by Africans on their immediate reaction to the war. Early postwar political movements in Kenya stressed the lessons they had learned when they observed different types of Europeans who were as helpless as they were themselves in the face of death and pain. Gone was the myth of the magic power of the white man. They also learned from revolutionary movements in other countries that they must rely on their own action to stand up for their rights.[7] In DOA we do not seem to have official records of African dissent between 1914 and 1918.[8] The case of Chilembwe in neighboring Nyasaland was an isolated attempt at resistance during the war. In an anti-war memorandum he wrote, "we have been asked to shed our innocent blood in this world war.... A number of our people have already shed their blood, others have been crippled for the rest of their lives.... Will there be any good prospects for the natives after the war? Shall we be recognized as anybody in the interests of civilization and Christianity after the great struggle is ended?" He warned his fellow Africans not to participate in a cause which was not theirs saying, "Let the rich, the bankers, the nobility, the merchants, the farmers and landowners march into this war and kill each other."[9] Chilembwe, the leader of a separatist African Christian Church, was not successful. His appeal to his fellow black tribes to secure for the underdog his rightly deserved reward was premature in 1915. Seven years later Harry Thuku laid the foundation for an effective movement of protest when he attempted to set up the Young Kikuyu Association as a political party in Nairobi. During the war the choices were limited to either an acceptance of being drafted into an alien cause or trying to hide somewhere until the war was over.

How did the Africans survive the war? Dr. Max Taute, staff surgeon and later staff medical officer who accompanied Lettow Vorbeck throughout the war, reported on his impressions and experiences just one month after the signing of the Treaty of Versailles. When he presented a paper on "Medical Matters relating to the war in DOA, 1914–1918" at a meeting of the Association for Natural Science and Medicine in Tübingen in 1919,[10] he still had a reasonably vivid memory of the human aspects of the war. He described successful military operations as well as disappointing setbacks, he praised German inventiveness to keep the sick and wounded alive in spite of a shortage of medical supplies, and he pointed at the trauma suffered by man when tropical disease and war-caused illness and mutilation besieged the soldiers in DOA. But he did not give an impression of the state of mind of the African nor did he mention any attempts at resistance during the exacting campaigns in which porters, askari, and sanitary helpers endured great mental and physical pressure. He admitted that the endless wanderings about of the army imposed hardship on everyone's capacity of endurance but saw a great advantage in the flexibility of movement because new camps had to be set up so frequently that the older resting places could not become health hazards. By 1918, however, a critical shortage of medical auxiliaries forced the military leaders to abandon their seriously wounded men, leaving them in the bush with only a few attendants exposed to the dangers of attack by wild animals, to infection by malaria, possibly also sleeping sickness, dysentery, and famine. They could consider themselves lucky when they were captured by the enemy.

Great concern was caused by an increasing shortage of quinine, the lack of conventional dressing material for the wounded, and the shrinking supplies of medicine, especially in the case of dysentery. Only when the Germans were able to replenish their medical supplies through raids into Mozambique and Nyasaland, were the grave dangers temporarily relieved. The medical situation alone might have induced a military commander to surrender but Lettow Vorbeck continued to fight and imposed suffering and deprivations on Europeans and Africans alike. The Africans who formed the majority of the contingent suffered more severely than the others. Taute acknowledged the hardship which the long lines of marching porters had to endure when their columns extended over 30 kilometers and obstacles along the road forced them to stand fully loaded for periods at a time. Everybody's endurance was put to a supreme test.[11] Taute praised his European comrades and wrote of the Africans, "the sacrifices of our black auxiliary personnel, our sanitation askaris, and the sanitation boys must not be forgotten. Their diligent cooperation with the medical service has supported us, their courage in battle has saved many lives, and the memory of their exemplary loyalty and devotion will remain in our hearts for ever."[12] Lettow Vorbeck's exorbitant demands on his troops, endured with reluctance and tacit rejection, were criticized by some German officials. Dr. Meixner, director of the Medical Services at the start of the war, has been reported as opposed to Lettow's policy of ruthless continuation of the war.[13]

It is difficult to transcend the realm of the generalizations and to present an exact picture of what happened in medical respects during the war. Taute disclosed that "official reports and other written data [were]

---

[7] See for instance, Rossberg and Nottingham, *The Myth of Mau Mau*, chap. 1, A. J. Temu, *British Protestant Missions*, chap. 6, Robert Rothberg, *A Political History of Tropical Africa*.

[8] Dr. M. Taute, "Arztliches aus dem Kriege in Ostafrika, 1914–1918," *Archiv für Schiffs-und Tropenhygiene* (1919), p. 23.

[9] Rothberg, *A Political History*, pp. 311–312, Loth, *Griff nach Ostafrika*, pp. 28–30.

[10] Taute, *Archiv*, p. 532.

[11] *Ibid.*, p. 532.

[12] *Ibid.*, p. 554.

[13] Clyde, *Medical History*, p. 98.

almost completely missing. Our statistical data, and especially our scientific notes must be considered as definitely lost." The paper shortage resulted in a reduction of written communications.[14] Piecing together the bits of widely dispersed statistics the following picture emerges. The German military force consisted of 2,500 men, 200 of whom were white. In addition there were 2,500 police askari taken over from the civilian administration. During 1915 the force reached a peak of 16,000 Africans and 3,700 Europeans. When Lettow Vorbeck's force crossed the Rovuma River, it still had 300 Europeans and 1,500 Africans, and at the time of the armistice all that was left were 155 Europeans and 1,100 Africans.[15] Lettow Vorbeck estimated the combined opposing forces at 300,000 men under 146 generals which would mean that there were 100 enemy soldiers for every white and black German soldier.[16] In 1957 Lettow Vorbeck spoke of 8 million Africans in DOA of whom one-fourth served in his army in some capacity, either as askari, or as porters or as peasants growing the food for the army.[17] It seems that on the one hand Lettow Vorbeck wanted to show how much his small military force achieved, and on the other hand he emphasized that the entire African population supported his war.

Dr. Taute, staff surgeon from the beginning of the war and chief medical officer after Meixner's resignation in 1918, had access to the wartime documents. He reported in 1919 that the German army started out with sixty-three doctors and five veterinarians all of whom were Europeans. In addition there was an undetermined number of African medical auxiliaries in each company which might have amounted to forty-two if, as he said, each company had four medical auxiliaries.[18] After Lettow Vorbeck marched into Mozambique in 1918, only thirteen doctors were left and by mid-July, four months before the armistice, the forces had just six doctors at their disposal.[19]

Both sides were medically understaffed. Both had an almost insurmountable problem of transporting invalid and sick men from field ambulances to safer stations where they could be properly cared for. The British had great respect for the German medical service. They attributed its functioning, in spite of Lettow Vorbeck's hazardous kind of warfare, to an excellent discipline and great professionalism. But they overestimated the German capability as Taute's figures of six doctors by the middle of July, 1918, indicate. Smuts's belief that the Germans were "seemingly immune to all the diseases which were making the British operations so trying" was far from the truth.[20] Both sides suffered from a lack of transportation facilities.

The Germans, however, had the inner lines and their numbers were smaller. They could therefore rely on a number of small movable treatment stations or field ambulances and, if necessary, hand their casualties deliberately over to the British.

Dr. Deppe considered war in tropical DOA so unique that he prefaced his war memoirs with a brief summary of its characteristics. Among them were

1. the tropical climate with its difficult living conditions for every single person, particularly because of malaria, black water fever and undulating fever.
2. the nature of the country and its inhabitants.
3. transport facilities.
4. the distance from the home country and the impossibility to replace losses of European manpower and supplies such as medicine. . . .
5. the psychological impact of total isolation from home.[21]

Many of these factors apply only to the German troops who were cut off from contact with their home base. But the British found it equally difficult to overcome the ravages of death and illness in DOA in spite of their open lines of communication. Incapacitation through disease among the British was 31.4 to one for the troops and 140.8 to one for the followers.[22] Dr. Horace R. A. Philp who served as government medical officer during the war but was a missionary CSM doctor in peace time, has given us a stark picture of human destruction. The men of the Carrier Corps were believed to have died at the rate of 400 per month during part of the campaign. "Large numbers have died in base hospitals, on the roads and in the Reserves after reaching home. Further, the men left for active service well and fit. Those repatriated have returned mostly physically unfit, bringing with them diseases innumerable."[23]

The immediate aftermath of the war was felt severely by the Africans and their new British protectors in Tanganyika. In Iringa in the Southeast the death rate rose to 3 per cent in 1919. The chief medical officer reported that the influenza epidemic of 1918–1919 affected half of the population of Tanganyika and had caused more than 50,000 deaths.[24] How was the transition from German to British rule carried out under these circumstances and how did it affect the former German province?

Administratively, the fact that an organizational structure existed when the British moved into the province was a mixed blessing. To start from scratch would have been difficult during 1917–1918 when the British took control of the German colony whose system of government was dominated by a military-civilian hierarchy. After the changes in colonial government in 1901, 1906–1907, and 1912 which had established civilian control in all administrative offices, the colony

---

[14] Taute, p. 526.
[15] Deppe, *Um Ostafrika*, p. 160.
[16] *Ibid.*
[17] *Ibid.*
[18] Taute, p. 327.
[19] *Ibid.*, p. 354.
[20] Quoted in Clyde, *Medical History*, p. 67.

[21] Deppe, p. 159.
[22] Clyde, p. 72.
[23] KNA, File PC/CP4/1/1 Nairobi, Annual Report, Kenya Province, 1916–1917.
[24] TNA, 1919, and Clyde, *Medical History*, p. 109.

reverted to military control during the war. Uncertainty about the choice of a new structure of authority determined the British to keep the German substructure of administration until major political decisions on Tanganyika had been made.

The chronology of the transition period reflects the gradual phasing out of military transactions. The British take-over of Tanganyika occurred in stages between 1916 and 1920. By the end of 1916 all of DOA north of the Central Railway from Dar es Salaam in the east to Kigoma in the west was occupied and political officers were posted in the districts. By March, 1918, the districts south of the railroad were added to civilian rule while a few unsecured areas remained under military occupation. By January, 1919, Sir Horace Byatt who came to Tanganyika from a position as lieutenant governor of Malta and with previous experience in African Somaliland, became the civilian and military chief of the territory. After the ratification of the Treaty of Versailles, Britain became the administrator of Tanganyika Territory under a Mandate of the League of Nations in 1920. The British government was finally in a position to issue a Royal Commission which made Byatt governor and commander-in-chief of Tanganyika, the same position which Governor Schnee had held until 1916.[25]

Fundamental changes in administration and policy could not be expected during this period. Until 1918 Britain was preoccupied with military affairs. Between 1918 and 1920 sentiment against imperialism began to rise and public opinion in England became slowly but perceptibly concerned with the rights of the indigenous peoples in English colonies. The time had not yet arrived when the Africans themselves would be asked for their preference. But postwar colonial secretaries and the new governors began to plan in terms of the development of the Africans. Indirect rule and greater participation of the native population became the postwar objective. To reach this goal many incongruities must be overcome to make the changes work. Sir Horace Byatt, the first governor under the Mandate, may not have fully understood what he inherited from the Germans. German policy of centralization of power was very different in intent from the British postwar policy of indirect rule which was just then in the process of being formulated. In spite of the creation of communal responsibility for selected local expenses, German district commissioners were not independent decision-makers. As Rechenberg said in 1911, the district offices (*Bezirksämter*) were to use their share of local taxes in the interest of the Africans but this did not give them the green light to go ahead with development plans. They were to serve primarily in a negative function as buffers between the native community and the settlers who did not contribute to taxation.[26] In spite of a larger staff than the Germans had maintained in 1914 which would have permitted decentralization, Byatt did not make use of greater provincial self-administration.

The first post war governor was described by one of his senior officials as modest though not impressive but well intentioned. Recent scholars have blamed him for his failure to carry out the officially proposed move toward decentralization, a move considered necessary to strengthen local native authorities. He was blamed for having stunted growth by his inability to coordinate the policy of his district officials. Everyone did what he had practiced elsewhere and it must not be forgotten that the new district officials were taken from widely dispersed areas.[27] Byatt was also taken to task for having missed an opportunity to return a larger share of land to Africans when the German land holdings were expropriated. Of 479,154 hectares, declared former enemy property in 1922, only 12,000 acres were handed over to the Africans. The German-held land had never been fully used, as statistics of 1913 show. Of 542,124 hectares alienated by the German colonial government in 1913, in the Kilimanjaro-Meru area, only 106,229 acres were actually cultivated and of these only 56,753 acres carried crops.[28] A good opportunity was lost, perhaps not so much because of a lack of consideration for the African but because it took time for a colonial governor to adjust to the postwar changes in attitude. Byatt, like his successor Sir Donal Cameron in 1925, operated within the framework of a patronizing scheme of responsibility which assumed that the first steps of their wards must be taken slowly in order not to disorient them. Dundas believed that Byatt chose to keep the system of akidas when he assumed the governorship because he felt that the Africans needed time to recover slowly from the physical and mental strain of the war.[29] Specific issues of great importance for Tanganyika were shelved for the time being, among them African participation in the growing of coffee, cotton, sisal, and copra, as well as the regulation of labor recruitment on European farms and in government. The first two *Reports on Tanganyika Territory* for 1920 and 1922 show a lukewarm attitude in this respect. In 1920 the official report spoke of the governor's confidence that an adequate staff of 108 officials for 22 districts of carefully selected officers would represent a good start. Those who lacked sympathy, tact, imagination, and patience had been weeded out.[30] Emphasis was placed on developing the African people on their own lines. But nothing was said on how to pick up the uncompleted schemes interrupted by the war, such as health projects and the careful preparation of an indigenous system of

---

[25] Report on Tanganyika Territory from the Conclusion of the Armistice to the end of the War, Cmd. 1428, 1921, pp. 36–37.

[26] *Ibid.*, p. 37.
[27] Sir Charles Dundas, *African Crossroads*, p. 232.
[28] Charlotte Leubuscher, *Tanganyika Territory*, p. 29.
[29] Dundas, *African Crossroads*, p. 32.
[30] Report on Tanganyika Territory, Cmd. 1732, 1922, p. 5.

production. For four years anopheles and tsetse had spread, irrigation and drainage systems had decayed. African labor was needed to restore Tanganyika to what it had been in 1914 and the good will of the Africans was needed to do the job. Regarding labor the second *Report on Tanganyika Territory* of 1922 ruled out compulsory recruitment of labor for private enterprises. It permitted compulsory recruitment for government projects only under special conditions for roads and works of advantage to the community. And even in these cases "stringent conditions to safeguard the welfare of the workers" were laid down to protect the worker from acceptance of a contract which he could not understand or from serving more than six months without special authorization by the governor.[31] Some of these stipulations had also been on the books during the last years of the Rechenberg and Schnee administrations. The test of the new regulations depended on their enforcement. In DOA pressure by the settlers and other interest groups had often been successful in fending off government controls of private labor.

Sir Charles Dundas, the first secretary of native affairs in 1924, described African reaction to the change of masters as illustrated by the phrase "When two elephants fight, the grass will be trodden down" or more drastically stated, "a plague on both your houses."[32] The British themselves were influenced by conflicting attitudes toward the reorganization of DOA. Their own imperial experience was a major factor to which was added a reluctant admiration of some German achievements during the past twenty years. They stressed the inadequacy of the small number of German officials, only seventy-nine administrators in 1914 who were distributed over an area of 385,000 square miles. They criticized the delegation of local tribal affairs to akidas who served as a convenient short cut to maintain order among Africans but who could not do the work of more expensive officials. They praised the German system of native education which provided their lower level bureaucracy with Africans who were literate in Swahili. They rejected the harsh discipline which included corporal punishment against loafers, resisters and those who violated labor contracts.[33] They praised the medical services but judged the sanitary services as far below the standards introduced in neighboring East Africa and Uganda. They decided to keep some of the German institutions while building up their own reformed colonial postwar administration.[34]

After Byatt left in the spring of 1924, senior officials analyzed their criticism of his administration and formulated changes which might ease the transition to indirect rule. They complained about a lack of liaison between districts which had prevented the coordination of divergent views among the officials. This was serious at a time when the Territory was in the process of being cast into a new mold. Some officers favored economic development, others the reverse, some favored native courts, others preferred autocratic rule. And out of the unreconciled contrasting views, nothing but anarchy was bound to develop. The Conference went on record as favoring the establishment of provinces under provincial commissioners. Whereas Byatt had recommended to center the political staff in the Secretariat, the Conference wanted continuity of policy in the Provinces without overcentralization in the governor's office. Particular emphasis was placed on the creation of a secretary for native affairs who would be a member of the Executive Council, a point which indicated the serious intent to reform and rehabilitate African society.[35]

After his arrival in 1925, Governor Cameron accepted the major recommendations regarding the provincial commissioners and the creation of the office of secretary of native affairs. He also agreed to allow for decentralization but still wished to retain sufficient control to effect the changes toward indirect rule as he saw them. Basic to the concept of indirect rule was the strengthening of native tradition and custom, but not for the purpose of creating a separate African nation within a European-governed state. As he explained it in 1926, "The native living in a European community cannot always be kept in a servile state. The native community will eventually, whether it takes one century or two or three for this development, claim a share, and a large share, in the administration of the country under the only system which would then exist, that is a system of government based on European methods."[36] This statement clearly indicates that Cameron was interested in remaking the administration of African society within the structure of colonial government. He thereby necessarily encountered problems when the ideological basis of colonial policy conflicted with the new formula of indirect rule. Wishing to extend economic and political co-responsibility in local affairs to African chiefs and educated leaders, Cameron introduced two statutes which defined the powers of native authorities and freed native courts from dependence on the High Court of Tanganyika Territory.[37] A senior commissioner's report on native communities in 1926 indicates that Cameron's crusade for indirect rule was shared by many of his officials. Describing the efforts made in the Arusha district "to lead the tribesmen towards a fuller and better realization of their position in the state fabric," he added a warning.

---

[31] *Ibid.*, p. 10.
[32] Dundas, *African Crossroads,* p. 106.
[33] Report on Tanganyika Territory, 1920, Cmd. 1428, p. 31.
[34] *Ibid.*
[35] TNA File 7610/1 Institution of Provincial System of Administration, 1926, p. 208.
[36] TNA, File 8057, 1926, p. 2.
[37] Ralph Austen, *Northwestern Tanzania under German and British Rule,* p. 154.

We must not however for a moment imagine that we are at all near the summit of our ambitions as rulers, indeed the goal is very far off—if in sight at all, and only persistent endeavour and ceaseless watching and teaching will bring about the state of affairs we are aiming for—that is the ruling of the native by the native with ourselves as semi-detached guardians of African tribal affairs.[38]

Regardless of the motives, Cameron's rule helped to broaden the basis of elementary education which was an essential prerequisite for economic improvement.[39] The Cameron model in Tanganyika Territory between 1925 and 1931 was conducive to the improvement of medical services. It was fortunate that at this time the struggle against disease, and particularly for the control of tsetse, was carried on by a number of determined, and often quite single-minded, individuals whose stubbornness made matters difficult for administrators but nonetheless significant in medico-social respects.

Shortly after the British military occupation of northern DOA a civilian medical service was set up in 1918. Starting out on a small scale with one chief and four regular medical officers, it was able to add one senior sanitary officer before long who had the help of 15 native inspectors and 741 sanitary laborers.[40] In addition to these regular appointments, a number of temporary staff members moved in and out of the service. The civilian medical service was not attractive enough to draw the best young men into the professional medical work in Tanganyika Territory whose future, politically as well as economically, was uncertain. Some of the leading positions were filled by men who had intended to retire after the war, like Dr. J. B. Davey, Tanganyika's first postwar medical director, and a few younger men with a liking for untried situations. Besides, colonial policy was in a stage of transition, too, from nineteenth-century paternalism of the plantation economy variety to postwar standards of experimentation in medicine and science. Added to these uncertainties was an atmosphere of austerity when the victorious European Powers were troubled with labor demands at home and their inability to pay their war debts.

Under these circumstances Governor Byatt's reluctance to increase the medical staff in a war-devastated country was not in the best interest of medicine nor was it good for the African people who set their hopes on their new masters. A succession of medical officers used up their energies during the period of transition until a semblance of order began to emerge. Davey, the first peacetime permanently appointed medical officer in 1920,[41] described the hopeless condition in which he found Dar es Salaam. In a city as mosquito-infested and plague-prone as Dar, there were no provisions for clean water. Water tanks were next to septic tanks and anopheles were rampant. Medical officers of health for sanitary work were not available until the international status of the Territory had been clarified. Among the few who arrived in 1920, Dr. R. R. Scott[42] cleaned up the city almost single-handedly. Byatt's priorities were not medically oriented during this formative period. Since the medical service was in the organizational stage, it depended on the governor's proclamations for the regulations of its services in order to be able to function. Byatt issued them only reluctantly.[43] When the medical service was finally capable of functioning on a regular basis, many critical situations had to be dealt with, among them plague in the Singida district, malaria throughout most of the country, sleeping sickness in the lake district, and the generally weakened state of health of the population. The Tanganyika Medical Report for 1921 singled out the "appallingly high infant mortality" somewhere near three hundred per thousand.[44] For financial reasons, as the medical survey made by the East Africa Commission of 1924 pointed out, important native areas in the vast territory had been neglected during the first years of the Mandate. In Mwanza, for instance, only one medical officer served for three-quarters of a million Africans.[45] By the end of the twenties the medical services had adjusted their manpower needs to the demands and operated in a respectable way. A few of the highlights of these operations are given here to indicate the direction of the postwar British medical and social services in Tanganyika.

One of the serious problems after the British takeover was the occurrence of bubonic plague in Singida in 1920 and 1921 when the department was understaffed. Not only was the government asked to stamp out the epidemic once and for all but the cost was estimated at £200,000 over a five-year period. The senior sanitation officer's plea to disregard the economic factor for the sake of humanitarian considerations is far more interesting than an account of the measures taken to control the rat population, to educate the people, and to treat them clinically. He wrote to the chief medical officer, "economically, I take it, every native life, on an average, is worth to the State £20 per annum for 20 years. Say you lose 100 lives every year for five years from preventable disease. Then the capital machinery of state is damaged, according to my calculation . . . to the tune of £200,000. This is a dead loss of capital—just the same as if your invested funds had depreciated to that extent."[46] According to his calculations, the government would save £152,000

---

[38] TNA, 1733/1 Arusha Report 1925, p. 5.
[39] Ralph Austen, *Northwestern Tanzania under German and British Rule,* interpreted Cameron's major interest in political and administrative change as genuine but limited by his acceptance of the prevailing colonial structure.
[40] Cmd. 1428, 1921, pp. 90 and 92.
[41] Personal communication to author, August 18, 1964.

[42] Scott became director of medical services in 1935.
[43] Clyde, *Medical History,* p. 105.
[44] *Report of East Africa Commission,* p. 55.
[45] *Ibid.,* p. 59.
[46] TNA, 2730/1 Senior Sanitation Officer to Principal Medical Officer, 20 June, 1921.

by stamping out the epidemic. Far from reflecting a lack of compassion, the sanitation officer's economic argument is an indication of the desperate financial basis of the medical operations in 1922. They had a low priority compared with other administrative functions during the period of transition. Long-term plague control depended on more solid houses or huts and continued campaigns against rats, and this again depended on a larger staff which did not materialize until Dr. Shircore became the second chief medical officer in December of 1924. The fight against plague, malaria, and yaws led to the consideration of another problem, namely how to integrate the African into a native sanitary service.

In this respect Major Keane in Uganda had done the pioneering work. Immediately after the end of the war he proposed the use of African talent and skill through a broad program of technical education but it took at least five years before his ideas were accepted.[47] In 1924 Dr. Shircore budgeted for nineteen additional medical officers to his staff but he knew very well that this was only the first step toward an effective program of preventive medicine. He, therefore, immediately examined another step in the same direction. He sought the training of dispensers, dressers, and sanitary inspectors. He first thought of mission-trained youths from Nyasaland. But the numbers needed in Tanganyika far surpassed the few trained men in the Livingstonia Mission. He also preferred to train locally available dressers to work within their own tribes in order to overcome the problem of alienation on the part of the selected young men and to give them greater acceptance with their patients. Shircore had only fourteen African dispensers in 1924 and needed a minimum of two hundred.[48] In 1925 the annual report for Dodoma by the administrative officer indicated some progress. The staff had been increased and was able to give more medical attention to its people. In spite of it, malaria continued to give trouble because, as the report said, the Dodoma species of mosquito seemed to defy medical science. In other areas the doctor claimed victory. Yaws, small pox, and plague had not occurred in Singida since the last epidemic in 1922. He was, however, most impressed by the manner in which the tribesmen themselves made use of the medical facilities. The change in Dodoma was particularly noteworthy because the German retreat left a residue of famine which continued until 1920. Tribes were disorganized, parents had pawned their children for food, wives had left their husbands, and the Wagogo had fatalistically accepted the belief that a "malign fate was pursuing them."[49]

Governor Cameron contributed indirectly to the growth and the improvement of the medical service. His personal relationship with Chief Medical Officer Dr. Shircore was good. The governor trusted him and listened to his recommendations. The use of Africans in the medical service was compatible with Cameron's ideas about indirect rule. Favorable to the improvement of the medical services was also the return of the British economy to a more stable situation. Medical expenditure was permitted to rise from £79,261 in 1921 to £143,689 in 1925.[50]

The fight for the control of tsetse in Tanganyika during the postwar years illustrates still other aspects of the medical services.[51] The man who carried out the fight was Charles Francis Massy Swynnerton who had become the first director of game preservation in Tanganyika in 1919. In 1920 he began to write a series of memoranda, requests, and appeals to the Secretariat in Dar es Salaam, the Colonial Office in London, the bureaus of Tropical Disease, and the Imperial Bureau of Entomology to have his plan for the control of the fly accepted. In July, 1920, he strongly suggested that a sleeping sickness commission be set up in the Game Department because it could marshall the combined efforts of the entomologists, zoologists, geologists in addition to medical and veterinary experts whose coordinated action must be used in a well-planned operation against the vicious enemy, the species of tsetse responsible for human trypanosomiasis.[52] This became the approach to the scheme which the government adopted in the succeeding years. His passionate pleading with the Secretariat in Dar and the Colonial Office in London revealed his scientific and his personal concern. Less than four weeks after his first letter to the secretary in Dar he repeated his appeal in a still more persuasive way which deserves to be quoted to show his deep concern.

It is we [the Game Department] who are in closest touch and best able to cooperate with the other chief wanderers —the sportsmen, resident and visiting. We shall also be working in peculiarly close touch with all political and police officers and shall have scouts and trappers actually reporting to them when they are working in their districts. We have in our hands, as no one else could have, an extraordinarily fine basis for the organization of a great tsetse information system and I would undertake to organize and use it to its utmost capacity.

At first Swynnerton had to contend with Dr. Davey, the medical chief officer who saw the greatest danger

---

[47] Ann Beck, *History*, pp. 80–81, 201, 202.

[48] TNA, File 7859, 1925, "Reference Suggestions and Recommendations of the East Africa Commission by Director of Medical Services," pp. 1 and 2.

[49] TNA, File 1733/ Dodoma District, Annual Report, 1925, pp. 17 and 29–33.

[50] Beck, *History*, p. 224.

[51] In this chapter the campaign against sleeping sickness as such is not presented. Only those aspects are sketched here which influenced the general pattern of medico-social policy in Tanganyika between 1920 and 1930. For more recent presentation, see Ann Beck, *History*, chaps. 5 and 6; John McKelvey, *Man Against Tsetse*, pp. 135–154; Ralph Austen, *Northwestern Tanzania*, pp. 195–197; David Clyde, *Medical History*, pp. 122–126.

[52] TNA, File 2702/1 Swynnerton to Secretary of Administration, 14 July, 1920.

of transmission of the trypanosoma in the uncontrolled migration of game. He proposed to go to the root of the problem, cutting off the food supply of tsetse by isolating it from game and cattle. The elimination of the bush and the cultivation of areas formerly inhabited by the fly led him to his proposal of cultivating and civilizing the sparsely populated savannah to prevent the further advance of bush, and with it, the fly. Swynnerton advocated the thorough burning over of vast stretches of infested bush near the lakes to be followed later by an advance of cattle and people from congested areas. The advance was to proceed in stages, first cautiously to the margin of fly territory, and then, after gradually coalescing a series of villages, their agricultural production and their farming methods should be made more efficient. He proposed experimentation in the fly belt after thorough burning had killed as many flies as possible. In his scheme the medical officer would then be responsible for surveying the success after carefully checking the people and their cattle who participated in the pioneering scheme. A constant evaluation must accompany progress toward the ultimate goal, the total elimination of *Glossina morsitans*. George G. Bagshawe, the director of the Bureau for Tropical Diseases, and Guy Marshall, director of the Imperial Bureau of Entomology, recommended his scheme as reasonable and proposed its adoption in 1922. Swynnerton started his gigantic campaign in 1923 and continued, with variations, until his death in 1938.

Of particular importance during the early years of indirect rule and in the interest of the reorganization of tribal life was Swynnerton's total approach to tribal living and tribal relationships. To find out the types of villages which were most exposed to sleeping sickness, he made experiments comparing one set of huts in dense bush with another located at the end of the bush and a third one, a larger tribal village near the end of the clearing. The smallest amount of tsetse was found in the latter and he therefore recommended the reconstitution of villages after the burning.[53] He was aware of the revolutionary character of his experiments. He recommended, for instance, cattle grazing on an experimentally cleared strip and then enlargement of the clearing adding more cattle as needed while introducing at the same time economic crops and better plowing. This was to be accompanied by medical attention and efforts to increase the population. All this, he wrote in 1924, required "propaganda and education to secure the natives' full cooperation in all measures." He conceived of the concentration of the people in new villages as a great amelioration of the social condition of the bush natives.[54] Throughout his work he knew that the aid of the medical department was absolutely essential in the relocation of the population and the creation of better living conditions in their new villages. His enthusiasm and his single-mindedness of purpose, however, did not lessen his self-criticism. In 1926 he was not satisfied with the results of his campaign. The fly still advanced in the Dodoma and Arusha districts. The creation of a new permanent position of medical sleeping sickness officer in 1926 indicates the concern of the officials. Dr. Mac Lean, the first appointee, had a staff of doctors and bacteriologists as well as a combined consortium of doctors and scientists who carried on the battle against tsetse. The death rate from sleeping sickness in the fly area was estimated at 11,500 between 1922 and 1946.[55] Gradually the immediate threat of the extended sleeping sickness epidemic of the years 1924–1930 abated. It was followed by an administrative program of permanently supervised settlements. After 1955 the new drugs made future outbreaks of epidemic proportions unlikely. The disease, horrid as it was, strengthened the administration of medicine in Tanganyika.

The East Africa Commission appointed in 1924 to investigate the economy, social conditions, and labor in East Africa, including Tanganyika, throws additional light on medicine in Tanganyika during the early postwar years. Their analysis of fulfilled and unfulfilled tasks comes from the perspective of the outsider looking in. It was easier for them to criticize since they were not responsible to the Treasury and the Colonial Office and did not have to follow up their criticism with improvements. Its observations were correct in general. The Commission found that less than a twenty-fifth of the population was within the sphere of medical influence in Tanganyika, a very unsatisfactory situation. It was satisfied with a general change of attitude on the part of the officials. No longer did they think of medical staff solely in terms of Europeans. To be effective, however, new attitudes must be implemented by changes in economic policy. Such a statement brings to mind similar statements by the German officials before 1914. The Commission wrote, "the future of the country is dependent upon the care of the native population, the increase in its birthrate, and above all, the prevention and cure of disease."[56] It was admitted that malaria still took too large a toll of the population. African living conditions were not good and epidemics like influenza created more damage among Africans than among Europeans. The Commission took issue with the insufficient training of Africans as sanitary and medical orderlies. In Bukoba the Commission did not find a single European medical officer nor had there been one for years. They found the neglect of important native areas for economic reasons not justifiable.

The medical director of Tanganyika Territory responded to some of the criticisms and proposals. He

---

[53] McKelvey, p. 142.
[54] TNA, File 2702/II Swynnerton to Chief Secretary, March 17, 1924, pp. 8–10.
[55] McKelvey, p. 155; Beck, p. 119, 125. TNA, File 7859.
[56] East Africa Commission, p. 553.

wanted Africans to be trained but their training depended upon economic allocations in the medical budget. In 1924 he had fifty sanitary inspectors in the field and he expected to have three times that number in 1926. He had included an increase of the medical staff in the forthcoming budget requests. Governor Cameron's tone in his comment was slightly irritated. The points made by the Commission were not new. A system of medical examinations for contract labor had been introduced. He was for a native medical staff that would be better qualified than Europeans to prevent the transmission of epidemic and endemic diseases. Cameron, however, did not think much for the time being, of preparing Africans for positions as independent practitioners. Until the educational gap had been closed, even the gifted young men were not ready to rise beyond the work of medical assistants. It was not difficult to train young Africans as compounders and dispensers as long as they had a knowledge of English which was still rare after the relatively short period of British rule. Cameron also hinted that any evaluation of medical achievements in Tanganyika must bear in mind the economic resources of the imperial budget and the lag created by the war and its consequences. The governor was satisfied with the direction of his medical program within the limitations of colonial government which he himself, however, accepted as valid.[57]

In another area the critical comment of the East Africa Commission was fully justified. Very laudably, the Commission devoted one section to scientific research and the Amani Institute. It was indignant that, in spite of efforts by successive colonial secretaries, "this world-famous research institution is, for all practical purposes, lying derelict, its laboratories unoccupied, its costly apparatus dismantled, the living quarters deteriorating, the magnificent and priceless collection of books and scientific records and specimens unused."[58] They recommended to reopen the Institute at the earliest possible time with the financial support of the three British territories of Kenya, Uganda, and Tanganyika. Their suggestion was prophetic. Fifty years later, the East African Community is in charge of the Amani Institute on a cooperative basis.

The basic outline of medical development in Tanganyika was completed by 1930. Increases in staff continued until the depression of 1932. The medical and sanitary services were combined under one director. More attention was paid to the health of the indigenous population. The medical service had a new format, different from that of the German pre-1917 model. Planning for economic development on a large scale did not become an issue until World War II in spite of the enactment of the establishment of a development fund in 1929. Priority was given to the control of tropical disease, the training of Africans for intermediate positions in medicine, and the improvement of the general level of health through attention to nutrition. It was recognized that the medical services were an important link in the "chain of social services." After the social and human destruction of the First World War, one was satisfied to have at least prepared the basis for a new pattern of services. Comprehensive planning for the future of Tanganyika and the future of its medical services did not begin until 1938.

VIII. CONCLUDING ESSAY

The history of socio-medical policy in DOA raises a number of questions. They pertain to the substance and quality of the services, to their nature and to their role in the overall structure of colonial government. One may ask whether the medical department possessed sufficient autonomy to influence colonial policy at the risk of colonial priorities. Furthermore, comparing the German and British medical administrations in East Africa before 1918, one finds them often dissimilar in spite of the fact that they were based on essentially the same external conditions. The British East African Protectorate and German East Africa shared the same geographical and tropical character. Their colonial administrations were based on similar ideological premises. Sleeping sickness, for instance, forced both powers to set up concentrations for their African patients. The process of selection of sites for the camps and the organization of tribal life in them were not entirely the same. There was also a difference in dealing with the problem of labor and the introduction of health care for workers employed by larger companies. The record of historical events permits an evaluation of social policies which were strongly influenced by the necessities of medicine and science.

Medicine in DOA started on a small level. From a staff of two officers who were part of a military organization the services rose to a more prominent status with the appointment of a chief medical officer in 1891. Until the end the major obstacle to growth was due to budgets which were limited by what Berlin and Dar es Salaam considered essential. As late as 1905 a major part of the African population was left without medical protection. Even in 1914 the staff of seventy-nine doctors could not cover the whole area. On the other hand, special emergencies during epidemics were acted upon promptly and efficiently. Auxiliary staff was made available for them to deal with preventive measures. Money for emergencies was appropriated when needed. There were several reasons for prompt action in such cases. Foremost, of course, was the threat which unexplored and contagious diseases posed to the health of Europeans and Africans alike. There was also the humanitarian aspect of medicine. Apart from medical ethics which doctors adhered to, there was the firmly rooted conviction that western medicine represented an advanced civilization which ought to be made

---
[57] TNA, File 7859, 1925.
[58] East Africa Commission, p. 85.

available to all those who were not yet capable of helping themselves. Furthermore, the dispensing of medical care and relief from suffering was recommended by missions and by government as a means of gaining the confidence of the African peasants who remained aloof from contact with Europeans or showed hostility to approaches by strangers unknown to them. In time, a more purposeful medical service developed out of these considerations.

For many years the German medical service suffered from its dependence on the military which might set priorities not always in tune with civilian interpretations of what could and should be done for the masses of the people. Though debated for many years, the transfer of the medical services to civilian control did not take place until 1912. Advocates of a separate medical department were particularly concerned with the inflexibility of the military chain of command which prevented experimentation and stymied change, so essential to keep pace with the constant advances of biology, chemistry, zoology, and medicine during the first decade of the twentieth century.

Events beyond the control of government played a large role in bringing about changes. A major blessing in disguise was the often recurring deadly diseases which demanded experimentation and research. Whether scientists experimented with the tsetse fly or the physiological effect of quinine on men, with resistance to malaria in different heights or the relationship between nutrition and human growth and the causes of infant mortality among tribes, once the investigations had started, they could not be discontinued and often led to unforeseen conclusions which required action. Sanitation often became particularly irritating to a succession of governors between 1901 and 1914 because it required personnel, engineering, and constant supervision in order to be effective. The apostles of sanitation had fought for decades in England during the nineteenth century to make the new cities and the countryside safer from death caused by modern industry. Now a still more difficult struggle began for sanitarians when they applied their knowledge to tropical conditions. The science of sanitation went beyond Disraeli's identification of cleanliness with morality, and sanitary officers proved that the knowledge of tribal custom was as important as familiarity with engineering or the habits of anopheles. Sanitation was professionalized and spread into related areas.

In still another realm, the procurement of labor, the policy-makers at the centers of executive power and the officials in outlying districts were forced to reconsider their conventional interpretation of colonial government. The settlers' stubbornly maintained conviction that it was the duty of the colonial government to assist them in the recruiting of the manpower they thought they needed for their own economic survival led to an uninterrupted controversy with the governor's office in Dar es Salaam. The Colonial Economic Committee of prominent industrialists supported the demands of the settlers. Out of these controversies between planters, industrialists, officials, and the governor's Secretariat, there emerged a perennial issue called "the labor question" in which health played a leading role. At first the term was used loosely as a cover-up for disagreement on labor contracts, responsibility of private employers for the minimum welfare of their workers, the right of workers to seek litigation when conditions of contracts were disregarded. Gradually, the term was extended in scope over the years after 1907. By the end of the German period it included the African workers' right to be protected from exploitation and added specific stipulations on working conditions and health. Those who came to DOA in 1890 would never have anticipated the change in the re-thinking of the "labor question" which ultimately led to inquiries by health officials, anthropologists, and district commissioners on the condition of the workers. Discussions on labor, originally dominated by preconceived notions of the "innate idleness" of certain tribes was, in its later stages, concerned with the ability of the African to learn and adapt to western habits. But here again, as had happened earlier in matters of health, the social analyses led to some reforms without affecting colonial policy as a whole. Revisionist thinking regarding colonial government was historically not feasible before World War I.

The period of "enlightened colonialism" after 1910 [1] pointed in a new direction. Emphasis was placed on indigenous crops. The fallacy of making DOA a settler colony was officially abandoned, at least in theory. It would, however, have taken a governor of greater strength than Governor Schnee to translate the theory into practice. Dr. Ittameier, a missionary doctor, recommended in 1915 an aggressively creative social and medical policy toward the African people. Assuming that the economic survival of DOA depended on the survival of its peoples, he contended that all the influences which damaged national health must be removed. He regretted that interest in the condition of life among the various tribes was of very recent origin. He pointed an accusing finger at the wasteful exploitation of DOA's greatest resource, its people. Without trying to explain why medicine had failed to play a more pervasive role in improvement of life in Africa, he simply stated bluntly that government should have done more. It should have placed more than one or two doctors in every district. One doctor was simply not enough.[2] His was not the view of a disgruntled

---

[1] Although Governor Rechenberg started the reform policy, it was sabotaged by the European community prior to 1910.
[2] Carl Ittameier, *Abhandlungen aus dem Gebiet der Auslandskunde* (Hamburg, 1923). "Wissenschaftliche Beiträge zur Frage der Erhaltung und Vermehrung der Eingeborenen-Bevölkerung" 1: pp. 2, 3, 60, 61. See also above p. 33.

physician who lost his perspective in his isolation. It was the recognition that the medical service was unable to fulfill its goals with the means it was given to pursue them.

Recent appraisals of the German medical services in DOA have credited it with solid achievements. Richard Titmus, for instance, wrote that

during twenty-six years of [their] administration, the Germans laid the foundations of a hospital system which was to be developed during the more tranquil years of British administration after 1918. They built some twelve general hospitals . . . [and] established a sanatorium in the Usambara Mountains, a "lunatic asylum" at Lutindi, and provided leprosy segregation for over three thousand patients." [3]

The systematic training of Africans to supplement the medical service as auxiliaries was not yet done before 1918 although vaccination stations against small pox, blood examination centers under Koch's scheme, and the use of Africans in the testing of glands may be considered as forerunners of dispensaries.

An unexpected stimulant for the promoters of colonial medicine in German and British East Africa was nationalism, a very real phenomenon though not translatable into economic terms. Frequent statements in official and unofficial reports compared the German achievements with those of British medicine and treatment of labor. They were impressed by British agricultural experiments and their Botanical Museum in Calcutta, India. They always emphasized the shortness of their colonial experience as compared with that of the British and their intention to do better than their neighbors. Irked by reports of desertion of workers on German farms to the British Protectorate, they insisted that treatment by British employers was not better but merely less organized. They saw in the lack of discipline in the relations between employer and employee a great disservice to the respect which the indigenous population ought to have for the European. There was a strange contradiction between German emphasis on a common European purpose in East Africa and the anti-British remarks when they compared their institutions. German scientists contributed decisively to the success of DOA. Before Amani they worked in colonial laboratories and seem to have been handicapped by insufficient financing. Powerful institutions at home supported them, among them the Institute for Naval and Tropical Hygiene. Amani itself represents a monument to the German Public Health Service.

The transition from German rule to government under the British Mandate was not smooth. After the breakdown of normal conditions in DOA between 1914 and 1918, further delay occurred through lengthy negotiations in Versailles about the mandatory status of the former German colony. A serious disruption of curative and preventive medicine between 1918 and 1920 added to the rigidly curtailed medical activities under Lettow Vorbeck and created a frightening regression of the general conditions of well-being in Tanganyika. But it was more than a time gap which separated the two regimes. The break with the past represented by a number of major and minor revolutions in Europe made itself indirectly felt in colonial countries. In Tanganyika itself revolutionary change did not occur immediately because its people were neither ready nor sufficiently trained in 1920.

Perhaps the greatest departure from the past was the beginning of planning which started before Governor Cameron took office in 1925. However limited the choices were from which areas of development could be selected, goals were at least stated, among them "the amelioration of the social condition of the natives of East Africa, including improvement of health and economic development." [4] That the improvement of the health of the African must include his personal life was indicated by the co-equal status which the department of sanitation was given with the department of medicine from the outset. All districts were staffed with European medical officers, small stations had Indian compounders. The scheme was set in motion by 1926, the pattern, however, was now different from that of the German service. Priorities set for the medical service were indicative of "the revolt in the minds of medical and administrative officials . . . against conditions which they (felt) can, and ought to be, remedied." [5] This did not spell the end of colonialism. It was indicative, however, of a faint echo of the revolutionary thinking of the postwar era. During the last years before World War I, German administrators had begun to include the welfare of the indigenous population in their considerations. Their motivation was, however, primarily pragmatic. Postwar discussions of the plight of colonial peoples had an admixture of humanitarianism and pragmatism.

If postwar thinking had changed, was there a significant difference between methods used and moneys spent? Judging from rising budgets, the attitude toward social and medical expenditure had changed. While £79,261 was spent on medical services in 1921 the medical budget had risen to £274,715 in 1930. Expenditure for the control of sleeping sickness in the district of Shinyanga had risen from £300 in 1923 to £1,126 in 1928. The statements about the government's intention to improve the health of Africans were not just idle assertions of good intention.[6] Britain's experience with the control of sleeping sickness in

---

[3] Richard Titmus, *The Health Services of Tanganyika* (London, 1964), pp. 1 and 2.

[4] Command Paper, *Report of the East Africa Commission* (London, 1925), p. 3.

[5] *Ibid.*, p. 53.

[6] Tanganyika Territory, "Annual Medical Report for 1945" (Dar es Salaam, 1945).

Uganda before the war had enabled her to continue in Tanganyika after 1920 without having to go through a learning apprenticeship. New emphasis was placed on agricultural production under conditions as close to normal living as possible to avoid the stigma of having to live in segregated communities outside the pale of normal people. In another area great success was achieved by Dr. Shircore's campaign against yaws, a spirochetal disease which had a demoralizing effect on large numbers of people because it disfigured its victims. The use of an inexpensive bismuth preparation produced in Tanganyika made mass treatment possible. Its effect was twofold. The large number of cases treated, half a million by 1929, demonstrated the value of western medicine. But, perhaps, more important was the introduction of the principle of rural dispensaries. At their start they were nothing but first-aid posts equipped with simple medicaments at which yaws was treated by injection with bismuth. Because of the spectacular rate of immediate improvement, Africans visited the dispensaries voluntarily in large numbers.[7] Rural dispensaries became too popular too fast. They expanded more rapidly than native authorities were able to train the tribal dressers. Those to be trained as African district inspectors were to serve in their own districts to overcome local innate reluctance to accept changes from outsiders. The youths selected for training must at least have an elementary education but their number was small and dispensers were often underqualified for the paramedical services which they performed in their isolated outposts without supervision. The expansion of rural health centers would have required coordinated action by the departments of Education and Medical and Sanitary Services as well as support by the governor's office and the Treasury in London. It was clear by 1930 that dispensaries would become an ever more important factor in medicine in Tanganyika. The lean years of the 1930's blocked further rapid development.

Comparing the British medical services in Tanganyika after 1918 with those of the preceding German administration, the general postwar changes in attitudes must be considered. Would German medical policy have accepted an increase in African participation? Would pressure by settlers to maintain their economic gains at all costs have prevented such a trend? These questions must remain unanswered, even with the hindsight of the historian. Nevertheless, medical history taken as a constituent part of general history contributes essentially to the understanding and clarification of conflicting trends in colonial East Africa. Tropical epidemics were trend setters for revisions in social attitudes. Not only did they force doctors to pay attention to the inadequacies of living conditions but they also alerted district officers to press for improved care and to point at the dangers of undernourishment. In campaigns for the prevention of contagious disease, public health officials supported basic education for the peasants because they found that voluntary cooperation rather than coercion was the key to better health.

There are other examples. The vicious circle of cheap labor at any cost was not broken by Governor von Rechenberg's reorganization of labor recruitment but by the cold facts of labor inefficiency due to the weakened condition of the laborers. Even then, the medical profession did not bring about a change of social policy during the Rechenberg administration. This was not possible within the framework of colonial government, especially as long as the medical service was under the control of the military. By 1909, however, doctors attacked the grossly inadequate number of medical staff employed in the colony. They made the military bureaucracy responsible for failing to attract young talented men to the service and their status was changed.[8] It was a medical man in 1914 who blamed the declining birth rate among Africans on the unfavorable conditions under which they lived in the colony, especially their inadequately small land allotments and their status as laborers on European farms.[9] On the other hand, the medical profession avoided political action and hesitated to present petitions to the Colonial Office to get what they thought was necessary.[10] On the whole the struggle for health in East Africa under German rule was courageous and had an impact on its history.

---

[7] David F. Clyde, *History of the Medical Services of Tanganyika* (Dar es Salaam, 1962), pp. 113–115; Titmus, *The Health Services,* pp. 5 and 6; Tanganyika Territory, *Annual Report for the Medical Department* (Dar es Salaam, 1946), p. 5.

[8] Claus Schilling, "Uber den arztlichen Dienst in den deutschen Schutzgebieten," *Archiv fur Schiffs- und Tropenhygiene* (1909), p. 37.

[9] Carl Ittameier, *Abhandlungen* (Hamburg, 1923), p. 19.

[10] See, for instance, the debate on the creation of a tropical research institute in Tanganyika in 1909. See above p. 36.

APPENDIX

I. COMMENTS ON STATISTICS

Statistics on the African population in DOA during the colonial period are admittedly only approximate. German officials knew how to collect statistics as can be seen from those recorded for the white population which are precise, broken down by ethnic origin, profession, and major locations. In gathering statistics for Africans, however, diverse methods had to be used. In accessible villages the people were counted. In other areas they were estimated according to hut tax receipts or other criteria. In some cases educated guesses were made.

The following data listed by *Amtliche Jahresberichte* (1914) project an apparently regular growth rate.

AFRICAN POPULATION IN DOA

1899	1902	1906	1912	1913
5,406,000	6,647,000	7,055,000	7,495,800	7,642,200

Source: *Amtliche Jahresberichte* R Kol A (Berlin, 1914), p. 287.

The figure for 1910 was given as 6,000,000–9,000,000.

In the 1912 report for 1911 the semi-official *Kolonialhandbuch* stated that the population reported for 1911 appeared incorrect.

In 1914 the official *Amtliche Jahresberichte* wrote ". . . the actual movement of the total colored population, its decrease or increase, cannot be easily determined as long as exact counts cannot be made" (p. XIII).

STATISTICS ON TRADE

Data on import and export trade, as well as production in the several parts of DOA, are abundantly available. They show a steady increase in imports to DOA as well as exports from the colony. But this does not imply that the colonial administration was self-supporting.

Imports: Values in 1,000 M.

1901	1902	1903	1904	1905	1906	1907
1,511	8,858	11,188	14,339	17,655	25,153	23,806

1908	1909	1910	1911	1912	1913
25,787	33,806	38,659	45,892	50,309	53,359

Exports: Values in 1,000 M.

1901	1902	1903	1904	1905	1906	1907
4,623	5,283	7,054	8,951	9,950	10,995	12,500

1908	1909	1910	1911	1912	1913
10,874	13,120	20,805	22,438	31,418	35,551

II. SELECTED DOCUMENTS [1]

To give a more concrete understanding of the historical situation in Tanganyika between 1890 and 1914 a few documents have been selected here. The selection may appear as arbitrary and spotty. It refers to only two aspects of the period, the role of the communities in relation to their African population, and government policy toward disease and scientific research. It is not possible to present in this monograph an extensive documentary record of the history of the German colonial administration in DOA.

I. CORRESPONDENCE AND DECREES RELATING TO THE ESTABLISHMENT AND DISSOLUTION OF COMMUNAL ASSOCIATIONS, 1901–1909

The establishment of Communal Associations under local district councils gave local control over expenses for local improvements to the residents of the area. Originally introduced to expedite the execution of matters not functionally pertaining to the administrative sphere of the central bureaucracy in Dar es Salaam, it increased the power of European settlers in local policymaking. In theory Africans were declared eligible for representation on the district councils. The documents below show that Götzen changed his mind only two years after the decree had been enacted. He decided that Africans were not competent as yet to fulfill their task as councillors in community affairs.

R Kol A 798 Bl. 188–189
Governor Götzen to Foreign Office
Colonial Division, Dar es Salaam
December 28, 1903.

During negotiations in Berlin regarding the decree of March 29, 1901, relating to the establishment of Communal Associations in DOA . . . I, myself, supported the statement in para. 4, section 2, "The colored population of the district must be represented in the district council by at least one member." I based my position mainly on my conviction that some concession should be made to those who considered native participation in local affairs as an essential factor in their education in the German spirit, thereby contributing to the spread of German prestige and German influence.

After nearly three years during which the above decree has been in effect, it is clear that this attempt must be considered as a total failure. Although the most respected and the most intelligent representatives of the native population were assigned to the district councils, not a single one of them has ever been able to understand halfway what went on in the meetings he attended, not even to mention the meaning of budget proposals, accounts, etc. This was true even when the presiding official took the trouble to translate the negotiations held in German and to explain them. The purpose of native representation in district councils as envisaged by its advocates has thus never been achieved and will not be achieved in the foreseeable future.

[1] All translations from the German original by the author.

Besides, in districts with a larger German population which will have a more lively participation in communal and administrative matters, opposition by the German representatives to the colored representatives in the district council is likely to develop and appears to have led to the view that the administration cannot expect interest by European residents in the negotiations of the Council as long as a colored member was present. Since, however, the administration of the Protectorate should be concerned to enhance the lagging interest [of the settlers] and since the colored member is nothing but a puppet, I urge you to consider the question to contemplate the removal of paragraph 4. [Götzen does not propose complete suspension of the rule but suggests the following amendment] "The discussions of the District Council are to be conducted in German. Colored members can be represented in the Council only if their knowledge of German is sufficient to enable them to follow the negotiations. If such a representative of the colored population is not available in a district, his place can be taken by another representative of the German community or by a representative of the East African Protectorate."

In this way the colored population would be *de facto* excluded from representation in the Council for the next twenty years, avoiding the complete suspension of the above mentioned rules, a measure which would antagonize the friends and advocates of [black] representation.

The native population itself is so indolent that it will not even realize the withdrawal of the right of representation in the District Council.

(Signed)
Götzen.

Officials explained the dissolution of the Communal Associations in 1909 as a means to adjust the development of poorer districts to that of the richer communities with larger incomes since local development was financed through local resources. District councillors continued to represent districts but under the law of 1909 they could include in their budget local income as well as central government funds. Two excerpts below explain the advantages of the new decree.

R Kol A 799 Bl. 108, 109.
Decree by Imperial Chancellor relating to the dissolution of the Communal Associations in DOA.

... Paragraph 1: The Communal Associations in DOA are dissolved as of April 1, 1909. On that day their assets are to be transferred to the East African treasury which enters into the rights and obligations of the Communal Associations.

... Paragraph 3: The members of the district councils and their deputies will be appointed for two years upon recommendation of the presiding district official. They must be twenty-five years old, be German citizens or [European] residents in DOA. The various professions should be properly represented in the selection of members and deputies. The colored population must be represented in the district by at least one member. Blacks are, however, to be included only if their knowledge of the German language is sufficiently good to permit them to follow the council discussions. In the absence of qualified blacks non-blacks with proper qualifications can serve as representatives of the black population in the district.[2] ...

Issued for Chancellor.

[2] See Götzen's statement, p. 23.

R Kol A 799 Bl. 117, 118.
From Imperial Governor Count von Rechenberg to District Offices, Subdistricts, Tribal Offices and Military Districts: Circular Order.
Dated Dar es Salaam, 17 August, 1908.

The dissolution of the Communal Associations in the districts shall take place on April 1, 1909.

The Communal Associations, though quite successful, had a disadvantage because, owing to their judicial autonomy, the more poorly endowed localities were not equal to the richer ones. This disadvantage did not only affect the less-developed administrative districts but also those located between the heavily populated districts in the interior with larger receipts, and the coastal districts with larger commitments because they were the starting points to the interior and had a larger European population like their neighbors [in non-German territory]. Further, a considerable amount of money collected in the protectorate, though used for justifiable purposes, was entirely removed from the control of the auditors ... It seemed, therefore, appropriate, on the one hand to abolish the existing Communal Associations and, on the other hand, to extend the authority of the district officials in order to include them in the planning and determination of the necessary expenses, except those to be taken over by the central administration, such as salaries of European employees, expenses for customs offices, etc. ...

A list of towns, their communal receipts for 1907 and the budget assignments for 1909 shows generally increases in funds. A few selected examples follow.

District	Allotment for 1909 Rupees	Communal income 1907 Rupees
Bagamoyo	107,811	72,000
Bukoba	39,391	
Dar es Salaam	135,742	102,650
Kilwa	110,725	65,000
Moshi	107,084	48,960
Mwanza	145,474	172,150
Tabora	101,607	53,050

Of particular interest in the study of medicine and society in Tanganyika is the fact that the new appropriations for each locality included money for medical stations and expenses for welfare support. A total of rupees 82,570 was to be used for dispensaries, medical treatment, food, and the control of endemic disease.

The list of expenses budgeted for all areas points at two major changes of policy. Though maintaining the decentralization of administrative districts, more controls over fiscal and policy matters were set up in the governor's office. Governor Rechenberg presented something that might be called an antecedent of "colonial development plans" since the projected targets included communal salaries for all African employees, medical expenses for Africans, the maintenance of elementary and vocational schools, the maintenance of buildings, roads, sanitation, and the promotion of agriculture and cattle breeding. (R Kol A 799, Bl. 119, 120). Rechenberg's continued feud with the settlers did not lead to results by 1912 when he was forced to retire. But at least a plan for extended government support for medical care had been presented.

II. EXCERPTS FROM MEDICAL AND SCIENTIFIC REPORTS

A. Medical Reports by Robert Koch and Bernhard Nocht

In 1906 Professor Robert Koch was asked to advise the German government on the control of trypanosomiasis in DOA. Accepted in his field of medical bacteriology as one of the outstanding authorities, he also played a role in the preparation of strategy when plans were devised for the struggle against the major tropical diseases. His methods of treatment of malaria and trypanosomiasis were not always accepted with enthusiasm by doctors who had gained experience in the field through their contact with African patients.

Koch's report on his observations on Sese Island in Lake Victoria in 1906 reflects the hope he had for the control of sleeping sickness through treatment with atoxyl, a new arsenic preparation which, he felt, would do for sleeping sickness what quinine had done for malaria. He considered the drug as a breakthrough in spite of the damaging side effects experienced by patients. He was confident that sleeping sickness could be overcome.

Robert Koch to the President
Medical Association in Berlin
R Kol A 5895 Bl. 150
November 5, 1906

At the beginning I thought that hardly anything could be done about the disease by way of therapy and I thought that prophylaxis should be directed toward an avoidance of infection and the struggle against *Glossina palpalis*. That, however, has changed completely. It has become apparent that we have in atoxyl a weapon which appears to be a *specificum* against sleeping sickness, similar to quinine against malaria. In my [previous] report I deliberately reserved judgment regarding the curative effect of atoxyl. Since then, however, three weeks have passed and during this period our most severely affected patients, many of whom would probably be dead by now without atoxyl, have made such visible progress that the specific effect of the medicine cannot be doubted any more. In the use of atoxyl against sleeping sickness, however, everything now depends on organizing a method of treatment that can be applied on a mass basis to the natives. In this respect I believe to have made a lucky choice. At present we are treating some 900 patients although we must refuse many looking for help and must limit treatment to the severely sick. This can be done only because of the way in which we use atoxyl. In two to three months, I believe, we shall be able to finish the treatment of the majority of our sick patients. We must then, however, observe the patients for an equal period of time to see whether there are no relapses. Only after we are sure that recovery continues without relapses, the task can be considered as completed. That prophylaxis of the epidemic follows from the recovery of the sick, is self-evident.

If everything occurs, as I hope it will, our expedition would be completed within five to six months, altogether one year, since the beginning.

As I see from telegrams and newspapers, people are working on sleeping sickness and particularly its treatment with atoxyl in many places, and it may be expected that in the near future some results will be published. In view of this prospect it seems to me appropriate in order to secure the priority of such successes as are due to the achievement of the German expedition, to publish reports on its work in full, or at least on its most important aspects, and I am therefore requesting respectfully, if there are no objections, to publish them in a widely read medical journal. Further, to stress the need for speedy publication of the report I want to mention that the government of Uganda sent three of their doctors to us to study our establishment and our method of treatment and that they have decided thereupon to set up as soon as possible a number of stations for the atoxyl treatment of natives affected with sleeping sickness. It is inevitable that they, too, will be successful and will report on it as we do, and it would be very undesirable if these reports would reach the public before ours.

Dr. Bernhard Nocht, director of the *Institut für Schiffs-und Tropenhygiene* in Hamburg, visited East Africa in 1912 on an inspection trip to evaluate the quality of the malaria control program. His report, open-minded and objective, contains interesting observations. He did not only describe local conditions from the perspective of the tropical medical specialist but he also added his personal evaluation of the general condition of health of the population. The brief selection which follows does not do justice to Nocht's ability as an observer and scientist. But it shows that in spite of his respect for Robert Koch he did not always agree with the control programs introduced by him.

Report by Dr. Nocht on his official visit to DOA in 1911.
R Kol A 5892, Tasche, 101.

In Dar es Salaam, as in DOA, acceptance of Koch's method of treating malaria infected persons exclusively with quinine is in part responsible for not having sufficiently separated European dwellings from those of the natives. . . . The so-called Koch method of malaria control for Dar es Salaam has had some merit, to be sure, but it is not satisfactory if used exclusively, neither here nor anywhere else in populated places. Its prospects have been diminished at a time when the railway connects Dar es Salaam with the interior. It is, of course, utterly impossible that natives arriving daily in Dar es Salaam by train from the interior can have their blood examined. Nor is it possible that those who are found to have malaria parasites can be treated with quinine. Besides, from the very beginning the quininization of the population has met with difficulties in areas where most of the anopheles was to be found, namely in the outer districts and the surroundings of the city because that is where migrant people can be found.

Dr. Nocht suggested that other methods of mosquito control which had been tested and proved to be successful be applied with energy and perseverance.

In discussing the quality of the medical personnel he regretted that there were too few doctors for the vast territory to be taken care of.

For the preservation of the valuable possession in the colony, namely its native population, it is absolutely necessary to increase the number of doctors in the colony. The medical districts should be increased in numbers and reduced in size. They should be posted by two doctors, so that one doctor can always be traveling and visit everywhere in his district with his dispensary staff while the other doctor can remain in his hospital and in the district seat.

B. Research. Correspondence on the establishment of a deepwater aquarium in Dar es Salaam

This correspondence began in 1906 under Governor von Götzen and continued to 1909 when First Councillor W. Methner responded in the name of Governor Rechenberg. Letters, memoranda, and petitions were sent back and forth to get government support for scientific research on underwater marine life and related subjects in the Indian Ocean. Scientists and heads of academies pleaded in vain with ministers in Berlin to use the exceptional opportunity which an underwater laboratory and research institute would offer. But budget considerations ranked the project at the bottom of the list of priorities. A few excerpts from this correspondence may illustrate the "no frills" practical orientation of the Colonial Office which was willing to spend money on trypanosomiasis research but looked askance at something whose immediate practical results could not be guaranteed.

Dr. Carl Chun, Director of Deep Sea Expedition
to his Excellency, Secretary of State for the Interior
Leipzig, August 29, 1906
R Kol A 6208 Bl. 38, 39

The request to establish a biological marine station in DOA submitted by the Royal Society of Sciences in Göttingen is well known to me since, as presiding Secretary of the Leipzig Academy of Sciences, I had an opportunity to warmly support the request.

I should also like to point out that the matter has occupied the Colonial Council (*Kolonialrat*) whose member, Professor Hans Meyer of Leipzig, has warmly supported the project.

If the plan to establish a biological station in DOA was supported with approval by all representatives in the field of biology . . . , their support was based on considerations of national and scientific concern.

As for the former, it would be Germany that would seize the initiative to give expression to frequently made suggestions that a tropical marine station be set up. An attempt by the USA in the West Indies was thwarted by the unhealthy climate. Since then not a single country, not even England, has considered the establishment of such a station.

Regarding the scientific reasons, the Indian Ocean represents an area niggardly neglected up till now. . . . [The rich plant and animal life is described]. All the problems which marine stations in Europe and America attempt to solve would be helped [through research] in such a unique and promising tropical area, quite apart from the fact that the equatorial waters present a number of new problems to the scientist. It is by no means impossible that such a station may in time be able to approach purely practical problems.

May I also mention that fishing conditions of the East African coast are practically unknown to us. . . .

Signed
Dr. Carl Chun

After several years, negotiations finally reached the top level of the German Administration as another excerpt from a statement by Interior Secretary von Bethmann Hollweg shows.

Bethmann Hollweg, Secretary of State for the Interior
to Secretary of State, Imperial Colonial Office
Berlin, June 13, 1908
R Kol A 6206, Bl. 75

. . . Reference is made to the enclosed copy on the talks of your Excellency with the various advisors which show that you have reserved approval of funds for a biological station until such a time that a suitable referee can be hired who is professionally properly qualified and has the authority to introduce order and unity into the scientific service.

Will your Excellency please indicate to me, in view of the events, what changes in the outlined project are considered desirable.

Bethmann Hollweg

But the impassioned appeals in the name of science and practical usefulness were unsuccessful. The story came to an end in 1909.

Imperial Governor of DOA, Dar es Salaam
to Imperial Colonial Office, Berlin
Dar es Salaam, November 4, 1909
R Kol A 6208, Bl. 99

I beg the honor to announce to the Imperial Colonial Office that on September 1 I was forced to close the Deep Sea Aquarium established on September 1, 1905.

The lack of professional personnel to supervise and care for the Institute was the determining factor; neither public nor private means could be secured for the operation of the institute and the employment of a professional scientist.

As will be known to the Imperial Colonial Office, it was originally planned, in agreement with the staff of the East African station, to have a naval surgeon direct the institute at first while in the meantime trying to have professional specialists come out with the cooperation of interested scientific circles and with their financial support. But appeals to the Societies of Science in Leipzig and Göttingen, and to the Prussian Academy of Sciences, as well as to the Prussian Ministry of Culture have been unsuccessful. And when finally the Imperial Naval Office was unable to station permanently a biologically trained naval officer at the East African station, the direction of the station had to be entrusted to insufficiently trained personnel and its scientific value was lost.

Besides, there was a lack of sufficient funds. . . . The

Office of the Navy provided 1,500 M on March 18, 1905, for the construction of a workroom in the Aquarium. This sum to which the station added 450 M was exhausted in March, 1908, while private sources contributed 33,150 M. These sums were not even remotely sufficient to maintain the institute in a scientifically useful condition. The considerable contribution of fiscal support by the Protectorate alone would not, however, be justified in view of the relatively insignificant role of the institute, especially in view of the unavailability of such means.

. . . The building in which the Aquarium is housed will be converted into a dwelling for officials.

I respectfully request to inform the Imperial Naval Department of my action.

Signed for governor
Methner

BIBLIOGRAPHY

Since 1890 an enormous number of books have been published on Tanganyika under German rule. Three major periods can be distinguished. The first, between 1890 and 1919, was influenced by settlers, businessmen, and agents of companies with economic interests and by officials, scholars, and professional men. Only a fragment of the writings of this period will satisfy the search for information. The reader will, however, gain an impression of the attitudes, sentiments, and drives which motivated the earlier colonizers. The second period, 1919 to 1945, is rich in German revisionist writings preoccupied with one major goal. It sought to reestablish a favorable image of the German colonial record. After 1933 revisionism was abandoned in favor of a vociferous demand to restore Germany as a colonial power. The last period, beginning after World War II, produced a number of scholarly publications on German colonial East Africa which were primarily concerned with the economic and social factors of the colonial system and reflect the anti-imperialist critique of the postwar years. It also shows the deep ideological divisions of the writers. It appears that the historian of colonial Tankanyika is faced with a difficult task.

The historian's task is not made easier in his search for documentary evidence. The collection of German documents in the Tanzania National Archives, in spite of a good filing system, is incomplete. The German Bundesarchiv in Koblenz has sets of papers of former officials but lacks the documents of the Imperial Colonial Office. The bulk of documentary materials on administration, labor policy, and health matters is in the East German Archives in Potsdam on which most of the source material of this monograph is based.

This bibliography records the documents, published papers, and books which are cited in the text. It also lists a few others which have been used in the preparation of the monograph. For brief introductions to the scholarly literature on Tanganyika, see particularly the following: John Bridgeman and David Clarke, *German* 1965) and H. Pogge von Strandmann and Alison *Africa: A Select Annotated Bibliography* (Stanford, Smith, "Germany and British Perspectives" in: *Britain and Germany,* edited by Gifford and Louis (New Haven, 1967). The latter contains a guide to the German archival and official literature.

UNPUBLISHED SOURCES

I. Zentrales Staatsarchiv, Potsdam *

Ansiedlungen in Deutsch-Ostafrika	R Kol A 15, 16
Die eingeborenen Arbeiter in Deutsch-Ostafrika	R Kol A 118–122
Bezirksräte in Deutsch-Ostafrika	R Kol A 237
Bericht über eine vom 13.Juli bis 31.Oktober ausgeführte Dienstreise Dernburgs	R Kol A 300–303
Die Deutsch-Ostafrikanische Gesellschaft	R Kol A 366
Arbeiteranwerbegesellschaft m.b.H. 1908–1911	R Kol A 528
Deutsche Kolonialgesellschaft	R Kol A 595
Die Organisation der Verwaltung in Deutsch-Ostafrika	R Kol A 764
Die Bekämpfung der Hungersnöte in Deutsch-Ostafrika, 1899–1917	R Kol A 771
Die Kommunal Verwaltungen in Deutsch-Ostafrika	R Kol A 798–799
Gesundheitswesen, Sanitätswesen, Ärztliche Mission	R Kol A 1024–1026, 1029
Häuser und Hütten Kopfsteuer, 1904–1906	R Kol A 1055
Malaria und Schwarzwasserfieber, 1902–1903	R Kol A 5838
Studienreise des Generaloberarztes Prof. Dr. Steudel nach Ostafrika (und des Prof. Dr. Nocht), 1911–1914	R Kol A 5892, 5893
Die Schlafkrankheit in Deutsch-Ostafrika, 1903–1907	R Kol A 5895
Gesundheitsverhältnisse in Deutsch-Ostafrika, 1902–1915	R Kol A 5647
Gesundheitsverhältnisse in Deutsch-Ostafrika, 1900–1902	R Kol A 5757
Die Schlafkrankheit in Deutsch-Ostafrika in 1910	R Kol A 5903
Akten betreffend das Krankenhaus in Deutsch-Ostafrika, 1896–1897	R Kol A 5662
Wissenschaftliche Anstalten in Deutsch-Ostafrika, 1906–1914	R Kol A 6208
Die Kolonialpolitik Sr. Excellenz des Staatssekretars Dernburg	R Kol A 6398
Nachlass Pfeil	31, 33, 37, 42
Nachlass Berner	5, 8, 9, 10, 11

II. Tanzania National Archives, Dar es Salaam

German series used for this study:

Allgemeine Verfassung	G 1
Medizinalabteilung	G 5
Missions-und Schulwesen	G 9
Eisenbahn-Abteilung	G 12

III. Deutsches Bundesarchiv, Koblenz

Nachlass Solf
Nachlass Richthofen

PUBLISHED MATERIAL

IV. Official and Non-official Journals Published During the Colonial Period

Arbeiten aus dem Kaiserlichen Gesundgeitsamt (Publications of the Imperial Health Department), Berlin, 1894–.

---

* The abbreviations given are those of the Potsdam filing system.

R Kol A (Reichskolonialamt) followed by the number of the document. In the text references.
Bl (Blatt) indicates the pages of a particular document referred to.

From 1894 to 1903 it published the annual medical reports on East Africa.

Archiv für Schiffs- und Tropenhygiene (Archive for Naval and Tropical Hygiene) Leipzig, 1897–

Amtliche Jahresberichte (Official reports of the Colonial Office) Berlin, 1910.

Deutsches Kolonialblatt (German Colonial Paper) Official publication of Germany issued by the Colonial Department of the Foreign Office, 1890–1914. After 1901 it issued supplements on special issues.

Deutsche Kolonialzeitung (German Colonial Newspaper), Berlin, 1894–1919, published fortnightly at first, then weekly, by German Colonial Society.

Deutsche Medizinische Wochenschrift (German Medical Weekly).

Deutsch-Ostafrikanische Zeitung (German East Africa Newspaper) Dar es Salaam, 1899–1914. Founded by von Roy with private capital but supported by Governor von Liebert. Professed aim: to aid the settlers and to stand up for the rights of Germans in the colony.

Die deutschen Schutzgebiete in Afrika und Übersee, Amtliche Jahresberichte (The German Protectorates in Africa and Overseas).

Koloniale Monatsblätter. Zeitschrift für Kolonialpolitik, Kolonialrecht und Kolonialwirtschaft, Berlin 1899–1914 (Colonial Monthly Publication).

Koloniale Rundschau, Berlin, 1909–1943. Ernst Vohsen, editor.

Mitteilungen aus den deutschen Schutzgebieten, Berlin, 1888–1929 (Communications from the German Protectorates).

Deutsche Tropenhygienische Zeitschrift.

Der Tropenpflanzer, Zeitschrift für Tropische Landwirtschaft. Publication of the Colonial Economic Committee, Otto Warburg, ed. 1896.

V. Books and Articles

ARNING, WILHELM. 1919. *Vier Jahre Weltkrieg in Deutsch-Ostafrika* (Hanover).

—— 1936. *Deutsch-Ostafrika gestern und heute* (Berlin).

AUSTEN, RALPH. 1968. *Northwest Tanzania Under German and British Rule* (New Haven).

BALD, DETLEF and GERHILD. 1972. *Das Forschungsinstitut AMANI* (München).

BOELL, LUDWIG. 1951. *Die Operationen in Ost-Afrika. Weltkrieg 1914–1918* (Hamburg).

BRODE, HEINRICH. 1911. *British and German East Africa* (London).

COUPLAND, REGINALD. 1938. *East Africa and Its Invaders* (Oxford).

—— 1939. *The Exploitation of East Africa, 1856–1890* (London).

DECHER, MAXIMILIAN. 1932. *Afrikanisches und Allzu-Afrikanisches: Erlebtes und Erlaubtes in Deutsch-Ostafrika 1914–1917* (Leipzig).

DEPPE, LUDWIG. 1919. *Mit Lettow Vorbeck durch Afrika* (Berlin).

DERNBURG, BERNHARD. 1907. *Zielpunkte des deutschen Kolonialwesens* (Berlin).

DUNDAS, CHARLES. 1923. *A History of German East Africa* (Dar es Salaam).

—— 1955. *African Crossroads* (London).

ELIOT, CHARLES. 1905. *The East African Protectorate* (London).

GÖTZEN, GUSTAV ADOLF. 1909. *Deutsch-Ostafrika im Aufstand 1905–1906* (Berlin).

GREAT BRITAIN, GOVERNMENT. 1921. "Report on Tanganyika Territory from the conclusion of the Armistice to the end of 1920." Cmd 1428, 24 (London).

—— 1925. Report of the East Africa Commission (London Cmd 2387).

GUNZERT, THEODOR. 1929. "Eingeborenenverbände und Verwaltung Deutsch-Ostafrikas." *Koloniale Rundschau* (Berlin).

HILDEBRANDT, FRANZ. 1905. *Eine deutsche Militärstation im Innern Afrikas*.

ILIFFE, JOHN. 1969. *Tanganyika Under German Rule, 1905–1912* (Cambridge).

INGHAM, KENNETH. 1965. *A History of East Africa* (London).

ITTAMEIER, CARL, and HERMANN FELDMANN. 1923. "Die Erhaltung und Vermehrung der Eingeborenen-Bevölkerung." *Abhandlungen aus dem Gebiete der Auslandskunde* (Hamburg) 13: pp. 1–146.

KARSTEDT, OSKAR. 1938. *Der Weisse Kampf in Afrika* (Berlin).

KELTIE, J. SCOTT. 1893. *The Partition of Africa* (London).

LANGHELD, WILHELM. 1909. *Zwanzig Jahre in Deutschen Kolonien* (Berlin).

LETTOW-VORBECK, PAUL EMIL VON, 1919. *Um Vaterland und Kolonien: Ein Weckruf an die deutsche Nation* (Berlin).

—— 1921. *Meine Erinnerungen aus Ostafrika* (Leipzig).

—— 1932. *Was mir die Engländer über Ostafrika erzählten: Zwanglose Unterhalungen mit ehemaligen Gegnern* (Leipzig).

—— 1957. *East African Campaigns* (New York).

LEUBUSCHER, CHARLOTTE. 1944. *Tanganyika Territory* (Oxford).

LOTH, HEINRICH. 1968. *Griff nach Ostafrika* (Berlin).

METHNER, WILHELM. 1938. *Unter drei Gouverneuren: Sechzehn Jahre Dienst in deutschen Tropen* (Breslau).

MEYER, HANS HEINRICH JOSEPH, ed. 1909–1910. *Das deutsche Kolonialreich. Eine Länderkunde der deutschen Schutzgebiete* (Leipzig).

MÜLLER, FRANZ FERDINAND. 1959. *Deutschland-Zanzibar-Ostafrika: Geschichte einer deutschen Kolonialeroberung, 1884–1890* (Berlin).

OLIVER, ROLAND, and ANTHONY ATMORE. 1974. *Africa since 1800* (2nd ed., Cambridge).

OLIVER, ROLAND, and GERVAISE MATHEW. 1963. *History of East Africa* (Oxford).

REDECKER, DIETRICH. 1937. *Die Geschichte der Tagespresse Deutsch-Ostafrikas (1899–1916)* (Berlin).

SCHMIDT, ROCHUS. n.d. *Aus kolonialer Frühzeit* (Berlin).

—— 1892. *Geschichte des Araberaufstandes in Ostafrika* (Frankfurt/Oder).

SCHMIDT, ROCHUS, and C. V. PERBANDT and G. RICHELMANN. 1906. *Hermann von Wissmann, Deutschland's Grösster Afrikaner* (Berlin).

SCHNEE, HEINRICH. 1936. *Das Buch der Deutschen Kolonien* (Berlin).

—— 1941. *Die deutschen Kolonien vor, in und nach dem Weltkrieg* (Berlin).

—— 1964. *Als letzter Gouverneur in Deutsch-Ostafrika* (Heidelberg).

TANGANYIKA MINISTRY OF HEALTH. 1952. "Synoptic Review of Medical Services, Tanganyika Territory" (Dar es Salaam).

TITMUS, RICHARD. 1964. *The Health Services in Tanganyika* (London).

WISSMAN, HERMAN VON. 1889. *Unter deutscher Flagge quer durch Afrika von West nach Ost* (Berlin).

Verhandlungen des Deutschen Kolonialkongresses. 1910 and 1924. (Berlin).

ZACHE, HANS, ed. 1926. *Das deutsche Kolonialbuch* (Berlin).

INDEX

African, attitudes toward labor, 23–24; reaction to World War I, 39, 40; representation in District Councils, 23; performance in agriculture, 47

Amani, foundation of in 1902, 34–35; and East Africa Commission of 1924, 45; Dr. Wilhelm Solf on, in 1912, 37

Arab revolts against Germans, 8

Arbeiteranwerbegesellschaft (labor recruitment company), sponsored by government, 23–24

Arbeiterfrage (the labor problem) in DOA, discussed in Deutsche Kolonialzeitung, 22–23; DOAG and its attitude toward, 1893, 22

Arning, Dr., on African labor, 26; reaction to DKG, Hamburg Branch (1912), 30; bibliography, 56

Askari, in World War I, 38

Assessors, role of in German administration, 9

Atmore, Anthony, bibliography, 56

Atoxyl, used by Dr. Koch against sleeping sickness, 1906, 19, 52

Austen, Ralph, 42, 43, 56

Bald, Detlef, 34, 35, 56

Behr, Graf Felix, associate of Dr. Karl Peters in DOA, 1884, 7

Bell, Sir Hesketh, and sleeping sickness control in Uganda, 1906, 17

Berner, A. A., Privy Councillor, rapporteur for medical missions, 31

Bezirksamtmann, office of, 9, 41

Boell, Ludwig, adjutant to Lettow Vorbeck during World War I, author of book on the war, 38; on Lettow Vorbeck's strategy, 38; on African loyalty during the war, 38; bibliography, 56

Breuer, D., on sleeping sickness duty in Ujiji, 20

Bridgeman, John, 55

British evaluation of German colonial administration, 41; postwar policy, 41, *passim*; protectorate established in 1920, 41; sleeping sickness control after World War I, 44; take-over of DOA, 40–41

Bruce, Sir David and sleeping sickness, 17

Byatt, Sir Horace, appointed governor of Tanganyika, 1919, 41

Cameron, Sir Donald, governor of Tanganyika, 1925, 41; and reorganization of administration, 41

Castellani, Dr. Aldo, and sleeping sickness, 17

Chilembwe, John, of Nyasaland, organizer of revolt in 1915, 39

Chun, Dr. Carl, director of Deep Sea Expedition, report to secretary of the interior, 1906, 53

Clarke, David, bibliography on DOA, 55

Clyde, David, 10, 18, 39, 40, 44, 56

Colonial Medical Advisory Council suggested for DOA in 1913, 30

Colonial policy and labor, 22, *passim*

Communal Associations, dissolution of in 1908, 50–51

Communes (towns), and budget increases in 1907–1909, 51

Cook, Dr. Albert, 17

Coupland, Reginald, 5, 6, 56

Davey, Dr. John B., chief medical officer in Tanganyika, 1920, 43; and sleeping sickness, 44

Decher, Maximilian, on World War I, 37, 38, 56

Deppe, Ludwig, on World War I, 37, 38, 40, 56

Dernburg, Bernhard, Colonial Secretary, on health care for Africans, 6; on labor in DOA, 24, 25; on native policy, 37

Deutsche Kolonialgesellschaft (German Colonial Society, DKG) in DOA, 7; on expansion of medical services, 29

Deutscher Kolonialkongress, *Verhandlungen,* 56

Deutsch Ostafrika (DOA), administration of, 7; early history, 7–8

Deutsch Ostafrika Kompanie (German East Africa Company), 7

DOAG on labor, 29

Dundas, Sir Charles, on postwar administration in Tanzania, 41; as secretary of state for native affairs in Tanganyika, 41, 52

East African Commission, 1924, Cameron's response to, 45, 46; on medical services, 45, 46; Shircore's response to, 46

Eliot, Sir Charles, on African labor, 22, 56

"Enlightened colonialism," 47

Feldmann, Dr. Hermann, on Africans under German rule, 34

German attitude toward British medical services, 48

German Colonial Society (DKG), 29; Berlin branch of DKG, 1913, 30; Hamburg branch, 1912–1913, 30

German Economic Association, 1907 memorandum on labor, 26

German government and African labor, 27

Götzen, Count Adolf von, governor of DOA, 1901–1905, on Africans in District Councils, 23, 50, 51; appointed governor in DOA, 9; on development of communes, 23; on malaria, 16; bibliography, 56

Gunzert, Theodor, 56

Hansing, German trading company in Hamburg, 6

Hildebrandt, Franz, 56

Historical literature on DOA, review of, 55

Hollweg, Bethmann von, secretary of state, on biological research station, 1908, 53

Holzmann Company in DOA, and medical provisions for labor, 27–28

Iliffe, John, 13, 23, 56

Illaire, W. von St. Paul, 24; on Dernburg's labor policy, 25

Imperial chancellor's decree on dissolution of communal associations, 51

Indirect rule in Tanganyika, 42

"Innate idleness" of the native, 47

Ittameier, Dr. Carl, medical doctor of the Lutheran mission in Kilimanjaro, 1910, 33, 47, 49, 56

Jühlke, Dr. Karl, in DOA, 7

Karstedt, Oskar, on DOA, 7, 56; on quality of German personnel, 9

Keane, Major G. J., medical training program in Uganda, 44

Keltie, J. Scott, 56

Kirchner, Dr. (Berlin), on medical missions, 1908, 32

Kirk, Sir John, British consul in Zanzibar, 5

Kleine, Dr., head of sleeping sickness campaign in 1908, 20; retrospective opinion on sleeping sickness in DOA, 1941, 14

Koch, Robert, and malaria control in DOA, 1897–1898, 15, 16; medical report on sleeping sickness on Sese Island, 1906, 52; preparation of sleeping sickness expedition to DOA in 1908, 18; and sleeping sickness in 1903 and 1906, 20, *passim*

Kohlstock, Dr. P., in DOA, 12; on staff shortages, 12; with Wissmann expedition, 1896, 12

Koloniale Rundschau, 1910, article on the African indigenous community and the African's potential for achievement in agriculture, 29

König, Dr. Harry, article on medical missions, 1908, 32

Külz, Dr., government physician, on native policy, 36

Labor in DOA, a continuing problem (the labor question), 47, 22; evaluation of, for the German period, 27, 47; and hut tax, 22; statistics on labor in construction work, 1909–1914, 27

Lange, Friedrich, associate of Karl Peters, 1884, 7
Langheld, Lieutenant Wilhelm in DOA, 8
Lettow Vorbeck, Paul von, on African attitudes during World War I, 40; bibliography, 56; as commander in World War I, 38
Leubuscher, Charlotte, on land question in Tanganyika, 41; bibliography, 56
Loth, Heinrich, 56; on World War I in DOA, 37

McKelvey, John, 56; quoted on sleeping sickness in Tanganyika, 45
Maji Maji revolt in DOA, 23
Malaria in DOA, Governor von Götzen and malaria control in 1901, 16; and immunization of children, 16; Dr. Robert Koch and malaria, 15, 16; Dr. Heinrich Ollwig and malaria, 16; Dr. Otto Panse, 13, and in Tanga, 15; Dr. Plehn and malaria, 14, 15; a political issue under von Rechenberg, 17; prevention before 1900, 14; Ross and malaria, 14; theories on causes, 14
Marshall, Dr. Ernst, on native policy in 1924, 37
Mathew, Gervaise, 56
Medical missions, 30 ff; definition of mission doctors, 32; Dernburg on role of medical missions, 1907, 32; and government subsidies, 32, 33; in general, 32; Dr. Kirchner not in favor of support for, by Society for Tropical Medicine, 32; Lutheran mission in Moshi, 1907, 31; relations between government doctors and mission doctors, 31; shortage of doctors in general, 31
Medical officials in colonies, 29
Medical research, 35; planning for, 1909, 35, 36; Dr. Plehn's views on limitations of research institute, 36; Dr. Schilling on medical research institute, 36
Medical services in DOA, achievements after 1900, 29, 30; beginning of, 10; under Governor Byatt, 43; under Governor Cameron, 43; comparison between German and British Services, 46, 47; decree of 1912 for reorganization under civilian control, 13; evaluation, 1896 and 1909, 12; evaluation of achievements by doctors, 1910–1914, 36, 46, 47; increased budgets, 48; influence on, 5, 6; organization under the military, 10; quality of service, 29, 38, 48; relationship between government and missions, 31; in Tanganyika Territory, 43, 44; use of Africans in medical service, 44
Meixner, Dr. H. F. A., director of Medical Services in DOA, quoted on Lettow Vorbeck's policy, 39; report on sleeping sickness, 1910, 20
Methner, Wilhelm, Chief Secretary (DOA), on abandonment of deep water research in DOA, 1909, 53, 54

Meyer, Hans, professor in Leipzig, 53
Müller, Franz Ferdinand, 6, 8, 56

Native administration, Charles Dundas, secretary of native affairs in 1925, on, 42
Native policy, DOA, 37; Marshall, Ernst, senior staff physician, on, 37; missionaries and native policy, 37
Nocht, Dr. Bernhard, director of Institute for Tropical Hygiene, Hamburg, on doctors in DOA, 52; report on visit to DOA and malaria control, 52

Oliver, Roland, 56; quoted, 9
O'Swald, German trading company in Hamburg, 6
Owen, W. F., in Mombasa, 1824–1826, 6

Peters, Dr. Karl, founder of German Society for Colonization, 6; German conquistador, 6
Pfeil, Count Joachim, in DOA, 6
Plague in DOA, discussed as a social issue, 1909, 37; in Tanganyika, 1920 and 1921, 43, 44
Planning in medical services, 48
Plehn, Friedrich, controversy on malaria, 14, 16; on tropical research institute in DOA, 36
Pogge von Strandmann, H., bibliography on DOA, 55
Public health, and African labor, 27; after the war in Tanganyika, 41, 42; campaign against rats, 11; development of, 1907, 11; evaluation for entire period, 46; not included in advanced planning, 5, 6

Quinine during World War I, shortage of, 39

Rechenberg, Freiherr Albrecht von, governor of DOA, 1906–1911, 11, 13, 19; controls over fiscal matters, 51; on dissolution of communal associations, 1909, 51; on reorganization of labor recruitment, 24, *passim*
Redecker, Dietrich, 56
Reichskommissariat, represented by district commissioners in 1891, 9
Reports on Tanganyika Territory, 1920, 1922, 41, 46
Research, in medicine, before 1900, 11; in oceanography, 1906–1909, 53; throughout the German period, 47
Richelmann, G., lieutenant-colonel, quoted on Hermann von Wissmann, 10
Ross, Ronald, on malaria, 14, 15
Rossberg and Nottingham, on World War I, 39, note
Rothberg, Robert, quoted on Chilembwe, 39

Schilling, Claus, director of tropical medicine, Infectious Diseases Institute, Berlin, in discussion of Tropical Institute for Medical Research in DOA, 36, 49; on role of the doctor in Africa, 36; on separation of medical duties from missionary work, 36; on military control of medical service, 12
Schmidt, Rochus, 6, 56
Schnee, Heinrich, governor of DOA, 1912–1916, on World War I and strategy, 38; bibliography, 56
Schutzbrief (Imperial Charter) for Karl Peters in DOA, 1885, 7
Schutztruppe, also called Wissmanntruppe, 8; established by decree in 1889, 9, 10
Science, its impact on Tanganyika, 34
Scott, Dr. R. R., in Tanganyika medical service, 1920, 43
Shircore, Dr. J. O., chief medical officer under Cameron, 44, 45, 49
Sleeping sickness, and attitudes toward Africans, 19; British policy in Uganda, 17; campaign against, after 1920, 45, *passim*; Commission organized by Dr. Robert Koch, 18, *passim*; comparison of German and British policies of control, 22; evaluation of campaign against, 20; experiments with atoxyl, 19; organization of isolation camps, 19; results during German period, 21; Swynnerton's approach to the control of trypanosomiasis, 1923, 44–45
Smith, Alison, co-author of bibliography on DOA, 55
Solf, Dr. Wilhelm, secretary of state for the colonies, on Amani, 35; on the economic development of DOA, 26
Statistics on population in DOA, 50; on trade, 50
Steudel, Dr. Emil, senior surgeon general, on shortage of doctors in DOA, 1909, 31; on sleeping sickness expedition, 18
Stuhlmann, Dr. Franz, with Robert Koch on sleeping sickness expedition, 18
Swynnerton, Charles Francis Massey, fight against sleeping sickness in Tanganyika, 44, 45

Tanganyika, Cameron's theory of indirect rule, 42; control of tsetse after World War I, 44, 45; reorganization of administration after 1924, 42; synoptic review of medical services, 46, *passim*
Taute, Dr. Max, on medicine in Lettow Vorbeck's army, 39–40; on missing war records, 40; staff surgeon in Lettow Vorbeck's army, 34; on strength of Lettow Vorbeck's army, 40
Tetzlaff, Rainer, 22
Thuku, Harry, leader of protest movement in Kenya, 39
Titmus, Richard, on German medical service in DOA, 48; bibliography, 56
Tropical Institute for Medical Research, discussion on having it in DOA, 35–36

Vohsen, Ernst, on goals for the East African economy, 1891, 10

Volkens, Dr. D. G., professor and custodian of the Botanical Institute, Berlin, on scientific research in DOA, 35

Warburg, Dr. Otto, co-founder of KWK, and professor of botany, University of Berlin, on the need for scientific research, 34

Wissmann, Hermann von, appointment as commander of the Schutztruppe, 10; and medical problems, 10

World War I, 37, *passim*; comparison of German and British performance in, 40; death rate, 40; loyalty of Africans during, 38; impact of the war on post-war era, 40; literature on World War I in DOA, 37; missing war records, 40; special character of, Deppe quoted, 40; statistics on war, 40

Zache, Hans, 56
Zelewski, lieutenant von, 9
Zupitzer, Dr. M., on plague in DOA, 11

MEMOIRS

OF THE

AMERICAN PHILOSOPHICAL SOCIETY

The Anschluss Movement in Austria and Germany, 1918–1919, and the Paris Peace Conference. ALFRED D. LOW.
Vol. 103.   xiv, 495 pp., 4 figs., 4 maps, 1974.   Paper. $8.00.

Studies in Pre-Vesalian Anatomy: Biography, Translations, Documents.   L. R. LIND.
Vol. 104.   xiv, 344 pp., 54 figs., 1975. $18.00.

A Kind of Power: The Shakespeare–Dickens Analogy.   ALFRED B. HARBAGE.   Jayne Lectures for 1974.
Vol. 105.   x, 78 pp., 1975. $4.00.

A Venetian Family and Its Fortune, 1500–1900: The Donà and the Conservation of Their Wealth.   JAMES C. DAVIS.
Vol. 106.   xvi, 189 pp., 18 figs., 1975. $6.50.

Academica: Plato, Philip of Opus, and the Pseudo–Platonic Epinomis.   LEONARDO TARÁN
Vol. 107.   viii, 417 pp., 1975. $20.00.

The Roman Catholic Church and the Creation of the Modern Irish State, 1878–1886.   EMMET LARKIN.
Vol. 108.   xiv, 412 pp., 2 figs., 1 map, 1975.   Paper. $7.50.

Science and the Ante-Bellum American College.   STANLEY M. GURALNICK.
Vol. 109.   xiv, 227 pp., 1975.   Paper. $5.00.

Hilary Abner Herbert: A Southerner Returns to the Union.   HUGH B. HAMMETT.
Vol. 110.   xvi, 264 pp., 20 figs., 1976.   Paper. $5.00.

Census of the Exact Sciences in Sanskrit.   Series A, Volume 3.   DAVID PINGREE.
Vol. 111.   vi, 208 pp., 1976.   Paper. $15.00.

Cyriacus of Ancona's Journeys in the Propontis and the Northern Aegean, 1444–1445.   EDWARD W. BODNAR and CHARLES MITCHELL.
Vol. 112.   viii, 90 pp., 24 figs., 1976.   Paper. $6.00.

The Autobiography of John Fitch.   Edited by FRANK D. PRAGER.
Vol. 113.   viii, 215 pp., 15 figs., 1976.   Paper. $7.00.

The Papacy and the Levant (1204–1571).   Volume I.   The Thirteenth and Fourteenth Centuries.   KENNETH M. SETTON.
Vol. 114.   x, 512 pp., 1976. $30.00.

The Letters of Lafayette to Washington, 1777–1799.   Second Printing revised and edited by LOUIS GOTTSCHALK and SHIRLEY A. BILL.
Vol. 115.   xlii, 437 pp.   1976.

Royal Taxation in Fourteenth-century France: The Captivity and Ransom of John II, 1356–1370.   JOHN BELL HENNEMAN.
Vol. 116.   xiv, 338 pp., 1976. $12.00.

Archimedes in the Middle Ages.   Volume Two: The Translations from the Greek by William of Moerbeke.   MARSHALL CLAGETT.
Vol. 117 (in 2 books).   xiv, 698 pp., 2 pls., 51 pp. of figs.   1976. $40.00.

Aspects of American Liberty: Philosophical, Historical, and Political.
Vol. 118.   viii, 233 pp., 13 figs.   1977.

TRANSACTIONS

OF THE

AMERICAN PHILOSOPHICAL SOCIETY

Distractions of Peace During War: The Lloyd George Government's Reactions to Woodrow Wilson, December, 1916–November, 1918. STERLING J. KERNEK.
Vol. 65, pt. 2, 117 pp., 1975 $6.00.

Classification and Development of North American Indian Cultures: A Statistical Analysis of the Driver-Massey Sample. HAROLD E. DRIVER and JAMES L. COFFIN.
Vol. 65, pt. 3, 120 pp., 12 figs., 5 maps, 1975. $7.00.

The Flight of Birds. CRAWFORD H. GREENEWALT.
Vol. 65, pt. 4, 67 pp., 41 figs., 1 pl., 1975. $7.00.

A Guide to Francis Galton's English Men of Science. VICTOR L. HILTS.
Vol. 65, pt. 5, 85 pp., 6 figs., 1975. $5.00.

Justice in Medieval Russia: Muscovite Judgment Charters (*Pravye Gramoty*) of the Fifteenth and Sixteenth Centuries. ANN M. KLEIMOLA.
Vol. 65, pt. 6, 93 pp., 1975. $5.00.

The Sculpture of Taras. JOSEPH COLEMAN CARTER.
Vol. 65, pt. 7, 196 pp., 72 pls., 2 maps, 1975. $18.00.

The Franciscans in South Germany, 1400–1530: Reform and Revolution. PAUL L. NYHUS.
Vol. 65, pt. 8, 47 pp., 1975. $3.00.

The German Center Party, 1800–1906. JOHN K. ZEENDER.
Vol. 66, pt. 1, 125 pp., 2 figs., 1976. $7.50.

Perugia, 1260–1340: Conflict and Change in a Medieval Italian Urban Society. SARAH RUBIN BLANSHEI.
Vol. 66, pt. 2, 128 pp., 2 maps, 1976. $8.50.

Crystals and Compounds: Molecular Structure and Composition in Nineteenth-century French Science. SEYMOUR H. MAUSKOPF.
Vol. 66, pt. 3, 82 pp., 4 figs., 1976. $4.50.

The Bourgeois Democrats of Weimar Germany. ROBERT A. POIS.
Vol. 66, pt. 4, 117 pp., 1976. $6.00.

The Presecution of Peter Olivi. DAVID BURR.
Vol. 66, pt. 5, 98 pp., 1976. $6.00.

Gaetano Filangieri and His *Science of Legislation*. MARCELLO MAESTRO.
Vol. 66, pt. 6, 76 pp., 4 figs. 1976. $6.00.

Recurrent Themes and Sequences in North American Indian-European Culture Contact. EDWARD McM. LARRABEE.
Vol. 66, pt. 7, 52 pp., 6 figs., 3 maps, 1976. $6.00.

Crown and Commonwealth: A Study in the Official Elizabethan Doctrine of the Prince. EDWARD O. SMITH, JR.
Vol. 66, pt. 8, 51 pp., 1976. $6.00.

Etienne-Denis Pasquier: The Last Chancellor of France. JAMES K. KIESWETTER.
Vol. 67, pt. 1, 190 pp., 1 fig., 1977. $15.00.

The Lonaconing Journals: The Founding of a Coal and Iron Community, 1837-1840. KATHERINE A. HARVEY.
Vol. 67, pt. 2, 78 pp., 15 figs., 1977. $7.50.

The American Philosophical Society

The publications of the American Philosophical Society consist of PROCEEDINGS, TRANSACTIONS, MEMOIRS, and YEAR BOOK.

THE PROCEEDINGS contains papers which have been read before the Society in addition to other papers which have been accepted for publication by the Committee on Publications. In accordance with the present policy one volume is issued each year, consisting of six bimonthly numbers, and the price is $10.00 net per volume.

THE TRANSACTIONS, the oldest scholarly journal in America, was started in 1769 and is quarto size. In accordance with the present policy each annual volume is a collection of monographs, each issued as a part. The current annual subscription price is $25.00 net per volume. Individual copies of the TRANSACTIONS are offered for sale.

Each volume of the MEMOIRS is published as a book. The titles cover the various fields of learning; most of the recent volumes have been historical. The price of each volume is determined by its size and character.

The YEAR BOOK is of considerable interest to scholars because of the reports on grants for research and to libraries for this reason and because of the section dealing with the acquisitions of the Library. In addition it contains the Charter and Laws, and lists of members, and reports of committees and meetings. The YEAR BOOK is published about April 1 for the preceding calendar year. The current price is $5.00.

An author desiring to submit a manuscript for publication should send it to the Editor, George W. Corner, American Philosophical Society, 104 South Fifth Street, Philadelphia, Pa. 19106.

TRANSACTIONS OF THE
AMERICAN PHILOSOPHICAL SOCIETY
HELD AT PHILADELPHIA
FOR PROMOTING USEFUL KNOWLEDGE

VOLUME 67, PART 3 · 1977

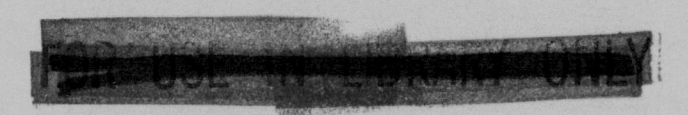

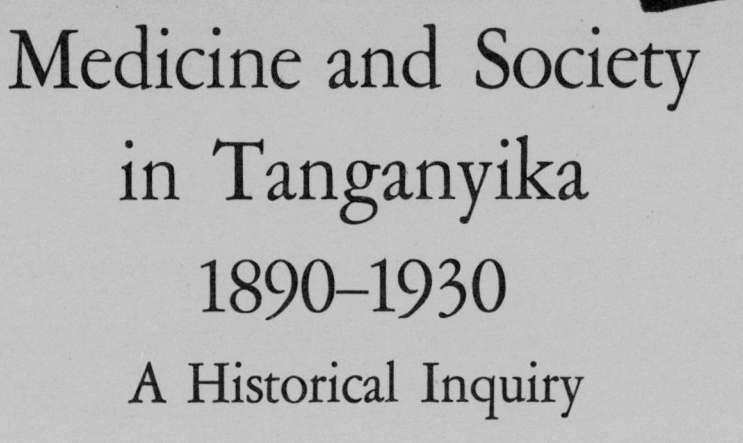

Medicine and Society in Tanganyika 1890–1930

A Historical Inquiry

ANN BECK

PROFESSOR EMERITUS OF HISTORY, UNIVERSITY OF HARTFORD

THE AMERICAN PHILOSOPHICAL SOCIETY

INDEPENDENCE SQUARE: PHILADELPHIA

April, 1977

PUBLICATIONS

OF

The American Philosophical Society

The publications of the American Philosophical Society consist of PROCEEDINGS, TRANSACTIONS, MEMOIRS, and YEAR BOOK.

THE PROCEEDINGS contains papers which have been read before the Society in addition to other papers which have been accepted for publication by the Committee on Publications. In accordance with the present policy one volume is issued each year, consisting of six bimonthly numbers, and the price is $10.00 net per volume.

THE TRANSACTIONS, the oldest scholarly journal in America, was started in 1769 and is quarto size. In accordance with the present policy each annual volume is a collection of monographs, each issued as a part. The current annual subscription price is $25.00 net per volume. Individual copies of the TRANSACTIONS are offered for sale.

Each volume of the MEMOIRS is published as a book. The titles cover the various fields of learning; most of the recent volumes have been historical. The price of each volume is determined by its size and character.

The YEAR BOOK is of considerable interest to scholars because of the reports on grants for research and to libraries for this reason and because of the section dealing with the acquisitions of the Library. In addition it contains the Charter and Laws, and lists of members, and reports of committees and meetings. The YEAR BOOK is published about April 1 for the preceding calendar year. The current price is $5.00.

An author desiring to submit a manuscript for publication should send it to the Editor, George W. Corner, American Philosophical Society, 104 South Fifth Street, Philadelphia, Pa. 19106.

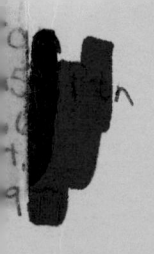

TRANSACTIONS OF THE
AMERICAN PHILOSOPHICAL SOCIETY
HELD AT PHILADELPHIA
FOR PROMOTING USEFUL KNOWLEDGE

VOLUME 67, PART 3 · 1977

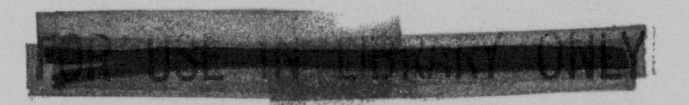

Medicine and Society in Tanganyika 1890–1930

A Historical Inquiry

ANN BECK

PROFESSOR EMERITUS OF HISTORY, UNIVERSITY OF HARTFORD

WITHDRAWN

THE AMERICAN PHILOSOPHICAL SOCIETY

INDEPENDENCE SQUARE: PHILADELPHIA

April, 1977